FAT TO FIT AT FIFTY

FAT TO FIT AT FIFTY

Chris Zaremba

Chris Zaremba

Aug 2021.

Photograph on front cover and pages 76, 77, 80, 106, 112, 157, 159 and 182 by Simon Howard of SNHFOTO.

Photographs on pages 138, 139, 142 and left side 143 by Matt Marsh of Matt Marsh Photography.

Back cover author photograph by John Frye.

Contents

AUTHOR'S NOTES

In places in the text, I refer to a website or video that you may find relevant at that point by means of a small-numbered endnote reference. It's not vital for understanding for you to see it at that time. If you want to follow the link, you will find the references decoded in the last pages of the book. This approach saves interrupting the flow of the text, and also means all such links are listed together if you choose to see them later.

This edition includes a number of colour photographs, reproduced here in black & white. If you want to see the original colour versions, look at: www.bitly.com/ColourPhotos

I would be grateful if you could let me know of any errors in the text that you find, so I can correct them in a later edition. Please use my email (below) for that and feel free make any other relevant comments: Chris@FitnessOverFifty.co.uk

Introduction

As you will see from the front, my name is Chris Zaremba. You can call me Chris, now that we've been introduced.

Did you know that over 50% of the UK adult population is over fifty? And that an estimated 90% of the published written and video material on fitness is targeted at ages below that? Redressing that imbalance in part is probably a good enough reason on its own to create this book, but I can add further justification by telling my own fat-to-fit at over fifty story, plus giving advice and recommendations which you probably won't have seen elsewhere.

A little background to me first. I was born in south London back in 1956, which makes me 63. I'm not claiming to be the fittest person of that age in the country, or in my town, probably not even in my street. But what is unusual about me is that I spent most of the first fifty years of my life overweight or obese, unfit and apparently allergic to anything like exercise, and getting worse with each passing decade. At age fifty, however, I had a couple of very worrying meetings that changed my life. From these I realised that increasing my fitness levels and reducing my fatness levels would be critical to my future – to having a future, that is. It's the change I've made since turning fifty that makes my story worth telling, I believe.

I was expecting the journey from being obese to fit starting at fifty would be a miserable one, eating what I didn't like and hating any exercise I had to do. But the opposite was true; it became a joy – yes, including the food and exercise. That path took me from treating fitness as something I've deliberately avoided to becoming my passion, my mission and my business. People have told me that my story is worth relating; indeed, they have convinced me that it is important for me to pass that story on, so that as many people who today have the same physical and mental approaches to being overweight and underfit that I had can read it, relate to it, and start planning their own route to a fat-down, fit-up life ahead.

You can read about those two distressing meetings, and my life in the years that followed in Part One of the book – 'My Story'. That first half of this book is about me; it is my fitness autobiography. In that part, I describe how I changed myself from fat to fit at the age of fifty and what has happened in my life since that age to both further my own fitness levels, and promote a similar lifestyle in others in their second half-century.

The fact that someone so inherently inept at physical activity is able to make such changes gives me, I believe, the credibility to advise others how they could make similar transformations in themselves. My recommendations come not from a study of internet-sourced theory or text books; I'm basing them on my own experiences and research on myself. Giving you the knowledge, encouragement and confidence to make such a fat-to-fit change is the aim of Part Two of the book – 'Your Story'. Perhaps it's your first attempt at addressing the fit/fat balance, or maybe you have tried before and not succeeded – either way, Part Two can help you make a success of it once and for all.

I hope some of the joy I've found in fitness is contagious and spreads from me in Part One, to you in Part Two. My intention is not just to help you grow fitter and live a longer, happier, healthier life – but to go one step further and for you to discover that you enjoy the process of change too. I have a phrase I use (a lot) describing people making their moves towards increasing fitness at fifty and over: 'It will add years to your life, and life to your years'.

Others have found this to be true. I hope you do, as well.

PART ONE: MY STORY

1 – The Bad Old Days

Most of this book concerns my life during the last ten or so years. That is the part of my story that I hope you find interesting and is the reason you are reading Part One of this book. In the chapters that follow I describe the changes that occurred to me at age fifty, how and why they had an impact on me and what I've done since that time; how I came to embrace a fitness-centred lifestyle and why I believe that passing this message on to others of my age group and helping them to review and adopt my views as their own guidelines is the most important thing I can do for society as a whole, as well as for those people I interact with.

In this first chapter, however, I am going back to the vast majority of my life, the first fifty years. I think it helps to have an appreciation of my life in those first five decades to understand my motivation, inspiration and approach in the years that followed.

It would be an understatement to say that I was not a sporty kid. As an only child I didn't have any sibling rivalry to keep my fitness levels up (no punch ups over toys in our house) and my parents weren't sportspeople either. I don't recall seeing either of them run, ever.

My earliest memories of sports activities are on a cub camp in Kent in the early 1960's. Such camps were based around activity. There was an indoor swimming pool, football and cricket pitches and a roller-skating rink and I remember how bad I was at every single activity. Today my lack of ability would probably be addressed as dyspraxia, but back then it was just called 'clumsy'. I specifically remember one sportier fellow member of the pack asking me why I was so useless at games. On the football pitch I was given a defender's position as it was felt I could probably cause least embarrassment to the team there.

I think being bad at one activity made me assume I would be bad at the next and this compounded both at the cub camp and back at home. I went to that camp annually for about three years. I was absolutely convinced I would be rubbish at anything involving sport and – guess what – I managed to fulfil that prophecy. At the end of each camp there would be a social evening back at the home base at which parents were invited to listen as the scout leaders read aloud stories of what a great camp it had been and how their offspring had shone. I specifically remember the Akela of our pack giving me only one mention that final year: 'And all the time, Zaremba just sat by the boundary shooting down ducks with a cricket bat – typical!'. Everyone laughed, except me.

Move forward a few years to my high school, an all-boys grammar school located in South West London, which changed to a comprehensive high school during my time there. Sports and PE were taken seriously, with two sessions of PE per week in a hall at the school plus outdoor games afternoons every Wednesday. I don't remember much about the PE sessions, except that I didn't enjoy them and tried my hardest to find a way not to participate, but the games afternoons do bring back specific memories.

There was a strong focus on rugby in the winter months at the school. I hated the sport, even though I was a little taller than average and therefore given the role of a prop in the scrum by the games teacher. Out on the field, I dreaded the ball coming anywhere near me. I would work out which way and what speed to run to make it look a bit like I was trying, but somehow only reached the ball a second or so too late to prevent it being taken by someone else – of either team, I didn't care. Needless to say, I never made proper school competitive matches, just the Wednesday afternoon run-around.

Two rugby-related instances remain firmly lodged in my brain from half a century ago. I can picture vividly specific minutes and events from those days as I write this, even after all these years. Firstly, there was the usual practice of the teacher identifying the two best players and making them team captains. The captains would then select the rest of their teams from all of the available boys, choosing alternately. And as I was always the last, I didn't actually need to be picked. As the only boy remaining, I was allocated to whichever team was next in turn to choose. However, on this one occasion, as I strolled over to the team that as last boy I would default to, the team captain exclaimed 'Oh Sir, can they have Zaremba? We had him last week!'.

The second was when both teams agreed in advance that I would not only pick up the ball in play but actually score a try, and kept this plan a secret from me. Somehow, in mid game, I was able to pick the ball up before anyone else. I then ran towards the goal with the ball, unable to believe I was doing it, but any observer would have spotted the lack of enthusiasm of the opposition and the way they just ran alongside without actually tackling me. I suspected something was up as I scored the try. This was confirmed when my captain said after I had grounded the ball: 'We thought we should let you do something right, just once in your life'. The captain allowed me to take the conversion, which I missed by a mile of course, and those three points for the try remain the only points I have ever scored in rugby.

In the summer term the school sport of choice turned to cricket. You won't be surprised to learn that I was equally unenthusiastic about participating. I can recall one incident from my only match I ever remember playing.

I found myself at the crease, probably last man in, and I can still see the bowler running towards me and unleashing a ball at what seemed (but I am sure wasn't) a truly wicked pace. Well aimed, it would have hit the stumps fair and square. My flailing with the bat did nothing useful, but I did prevent the ball meeting the stumps by leaving my ankle in the way. As a result, I had to limp off. I had to go off anyway as being out LBW. Sympathy there wasn't, but laughs aplenty from members of both teams and I remember a corker of a black bruise over that ankle. My cricketing life was over in its first over. I was never asked to bat again and that bruise kept me away from PE and games for several weeks. So, it wasn't all bad news.

Eventually I became more creative in finding excuses that meant I didn't need to go onto the sports fields at all, whether cricket or rugby. I am sure my hand-written pretend-parental notes requesting excusing from games or PE fooled no one, but generally the teachers couldn't be bothered to argue, so I could sit much of these events out. I was treated as an irrelevance by the teachers and as just being pathetic by my fellow pupils. I am sure that kids inept at sport are treated much better at school these days. I certainly hope so.

I wasn't the only non-sporty person in my year at school. I developed good friendships with Richard and Shawn, who equally ducked out of sporting activities in those days. Richard had a medical condition that kept him away and Shawn was a clever artful dodger in his own way. I learnt a few tricks from him. It helped that that the three of us shared an interest in railways and were able to chat away on that topic while others did all the exertion. I remember many chats between us about trains while watching other pupils from our year take Wednesday games much more seriously than any of us did. It helped that the school had a Railway Society (not uncommon in those days), and with the three of us being self-elected to the Committee we had an almost-legitimate reason to be chatting about trains rather than doing sport or exercise.

As we neared the top end of the school the three of us discovered an interest in beer and pubs and became early supporters of the Campaign for Real Ale. Adding other friends from younger years at school to our social group, such as Mike and Kevan, we soon travelled to just about every pub in the borough and many much further away. The distant trips combined both a chance to travel on rail and to sample local beers, a double tick. Girlfriends came and went and often joined us on those local pub trips and further afield. I remember many narrowboat holidays as an excellent way of linking pubs together. All activities which share a lack of exercise and an increased opportunity to experience low-quality nutrition, as I am sure you have noticed.

As sixth-form changed into full-time work for me, I seriously got into high-volume food of low nutritional value. I commuted to the City of London from Cheam, a northbound journey which included eating a bar of chocolate from the station newsagent for the morning train and a bacon sandwich on arrival at the office. Lunch was invariably something with chips in the staff canteen and a beer with new work colleagues, and then the journey home – usually another chocolate bar for the train and then either fish and chips or burger and chips on the short evening walk home from the station. And probably a beer or two with some of those aforementioned friends in the evening. Weekends were different – no commuting, of course, but more time with friends which so often was beer and pub-grub or fast-food enhanced. I was on first-name terms with all the staff at Cheam Superfish and I reckon I could have been top of the table in loyalty points at the American Way burger bar on Cheam Broadway if they had had such a scheme. You can imagine the result of all those less-than-perfectly healthy calories combined with very little activity.

After a few years of work, I went to university in Lancaster as a mature student – 'the most immature mature student I have ever met', according to my tutor. Here was an educational establishment that actually offered on-site beer and cheap fish and chips, and for which games and sport were totally optional. I also became interested in the University's own radio station – and quickly found myself in the role of presenting shows at times many students were involved in sport. That was another good way to ensure I didn't have to think too hard about the reasons why I dodged exercise. Another joy at Lancaster – the city and its surroundings had good ales on offer in wonderful pubs (it still has). Overall, an excellent way to spend three years.

While at Lancaster I discovered the game of squash, and found that I was actually not-totally-rubbish at it. In fact, I got hooked and my squash friend from those days, Tony, joins everybody else I've named so far in remaining a very good friend to this day. I now realise that one of the reasons that I loved squash (and similarly weight-training much later in my life) is that these are not team activities. I couldn't handle the team peer pressure in my earlier life as those tales from the rugby pitch show. Despite the passage of half-a-century I realise I still have the same hang-up. I avoid team sports today.

I stayed out of the bars long enough to earn a 2:2 degree in Computer Science, and re-joined the world of work. But I carried on consuming far more calories than I was using, eating (mainly the wrong things) and drinking (definitely the wrong things) for most of the following decades. I don't have records of how much a weighed in those days but I am sure that my average weight increased for every year from late teenage on.

I changed jobs and location a few times, but fitness was nowhere on my priority list. I found time to study and qualify for a flying licence so that I could rent a single engine plane and travel, a new hobby that, for a change, wasn't dominated by eating and drinking. Then at the end of 1995 I met Jenny, a lovely young lady that I dreamed would one day be my wife. We started 'going out' – I think that was the term used at that time – and I supported her massively in her sporting endeavours. Yes, she was into sport in a way that I wasn't and she loved her running, triathlons, football, hockey and more. I know she would have liked me to become fitter, to lose some weight, lose the substantial spare tyre that had built up around my belly, but I was having a great time and there was no way I would could live an active life like hers.

My dream of marriage came true at the start of 1999, and I recall that I did try and become slimmer for our wedding day photos. During the months prior to the big day, I lost around a stone (14lb, 6kg) in weight to take me down to 15stone 10lb (220lb, 100kg) so I looked more presentable for our photos. Had I been thinking more positively with a long-term view and less about trying to look better for a single day, that could have been the start of my fitness journey there and then. I had taken off that stone, admittedly probably the low-hanging fruit of my excess weight, but it certainly could have been a great initial kick-start to a fitter approach for the years to follow.

However, it wasn't, as I regained that lost weight. And then proceeded to add considerably more.

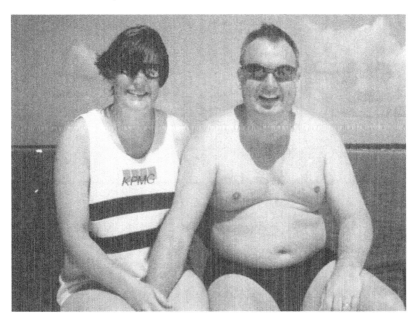

An early photo with Jenny with me almost at my fattest

I was still playing squash, very enthusiastically too. There was a small part of me that felt it was good to do something active, something that made me sweat a huge amount, an activity that didn't involve food and drink or simply sitting down watching TV with mindless eating to accompany it.

Hurtling around a squash court two or three times a week, bouncing off walls as a dripping mass is far from the optimal fitness activity for an obese bloke. I rather suspect you knew that already; it proved a shame that I didn't.

While unlikely to promote health in an excessively-overweight participant, such activity is likely to do virtually the opposite: cause injury. For me, that came as a total Achilles Tendon rupture during a game, without doubt caused by the extreme forces my heavy weight was putting through my calf and ankle as I thundered around the court.

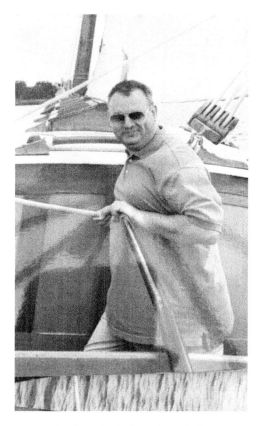

A couple of weeks before the Achilles injury

The surgeon suggested removing half of the tendon from the good foot and transplanting it to the injured one. I didn't like the sound of that, changing one bad foot into two, so I chose the alternative approach of a nine-month period in an orthopaedic boot while the tendon rebuilt itself.

This came with the warning that I was unlikely ever to run again, and would always have a limp when walking. The only thing that had been anything close to voluntary exercise in my life was over.

I was up to about 18 stone (252lb, 115kg) and a bodyfat percentage I estimate of 40%.

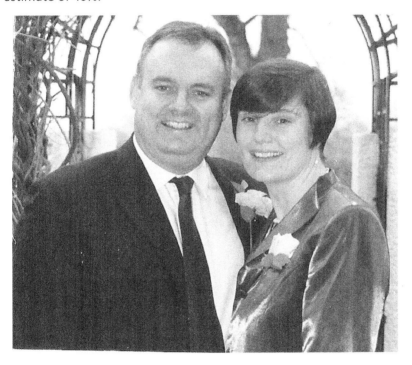

The heaviest person at Jenny's sister's wedding

The orthopaedic boot was off, I could walk without any pain, but by any definition, I was obese, an adjective confirmed by my BMI, which I have just calculated to have been 36 at that time, based on my height of 5' 10" (178cm).

If I had any sense in those days, I should have changed my ways in both nutrition and movement. It wasn't that I had decided that I would rather be obese than fit, it was that fitness was still way off my radar. As you now know, I had never been sporty, or active in any way, apart from those early days behaving like a lunatic on a squash court. Fitness was how other people spent some time, and sport was something to watch on TV.

You would think that spending time with a sports-keen wife would have resulted in something rubbing off on me; well, I agree – I would have thought that too. But it didn't.

A few months after my fiftieth birthday, visits to two separate doctors were to change my life.

2 – Motivation for Change

I was having a great time when I reached fifty. I had been married for seven years to a truly wonderful lady, had a good-ish job (almost a career) that paid well and gave me enough free time to travel where I wanted, ate whatever tempted me and drank whenever I could find a decent ale. I still had my friends from school, and they loved railways and traditional ale as much as I did. Nothing diminished there over the decades. It was a shame about having to drop the squash due to the Achilles Tendon injury, but I had mentally moved on from that and had recovered sufficiently that I could walk without noticing it. Life was good and, as they say, what could possibly go wrong?

Fitness and health were not matters of any concern to me. I wasn't deliberately ignoring them, or acting in a way to decrease or downgrade their significance in any way. It's just that these factors simply weren't things I ever thought about. Two incidents occurred, remarkably separated by only a few weeks, which were to lead to a major shift in my life. Without these incidents, this book would not have turned out the way it has and would certainly have needed a different title.

The first was a regular and routine visit I paid to a specialist doctor, one qualified to be an Aviation Medical Examiner and appointed to that role by the flying authority in the UK, the CAA. I've already mentioned that I had a recreational pilot's licence and you will not be surprised to hear that a medical exam needs to be passed in order to qualify, including for the small, single-engine aircraft, such as the ones I rented. Such a medical has to be renewed at intervals in order to continue the validity of the licence and, as the pilot gets older, the tests become more frequent and increasingly stringent.

This particular visit was at the start of 2007, a few months past my fiftieth birthday, which meant that the aviation medical was now annual for me. I went to the same Aviation Medical Examiner in central London that I had seen previously, expecting a routine similar to previous visits. However, there was a less-desired outcome this time. His conclusion at the end of his examination was that I had failed the medical. And that meant that I could no longer legally pilot a small plane. I could go with an instructor, but no longer fly as pilot-in-command of the aircraft on my own or with my wife or friends. It was like having L-plates reimposed on you once you're used to driving.

I failed in four specific areas – my height/weight ratio, blood pressure, bloodstream fats and blood sugars. The doctor said that none of my results in these showed an emergency situation. Indeed, had I been 49 he would have passed me as fit to remain a pilot. However, the results on all areas meant he had no option but to declare me medically unfit for that role, and therefore my licence to fly was revoked from that moment. His remit was specifically, of course, to check against the requirements of the medical and had no obligation to give advice; but he did so, and the guidance was that all of the measurements that had led to my examination failure could be improved if I lost some weight – nothing more specific than that – and that if I did that, he would welcome me back for another examination which he felt I would pass.

It was a blow to have to drop one of my hobbies, but not such a setback that I actually did anything about it. It was January. I did all my flying in the decent summer weather and I remember thinking that I had plenty of time to follow his advice and be re-tested before the flying season resumed for me a few months later. So, as I popped in for a pint or two at a nearby favourite pub after the exam – the Barley Mow in Dorset Street, Marylebone – I managed to mentally file this warning into the 'to be looked at later' part of my brain and I expected life to return to normal until thinking about it again in the spring.

The advice of that Aviation Medical Examiner was not uppermost in my mind when I went for a visit to my GP a few weeks later. I can't remember now what the reason for my visit to her was, probably something like athlete's foot or earwax, but it certainly wasn't linked to my weight or fitness. Having given me the treatment or advice I was seeking, the GP asked about any efforts I was making to lose weight, as she had observed my weight appeared to be increasing over the years that I had been on her books. I then mentioned the results of my aviation medical, which prompted her into stating that she now wanted to arrange her own full medical for me. I don't know to this day if she would have suggested this additional medical examination had I not mentioned the results of my aviation medical tests.

The tests undertaken included a repetition of the analyses that I had failed in my aviation medical examination, with more on top, such as lung function and aerobic capacity. The blood test was more thorough than for the aviation test, as it had to be performed at a local hospital and sent away for detailed investigation. I don't have a record of the specific numbers revealed in the test results. However, I do remember some of the words the doctor used in her summary from well over a decade ago with stunning clarity.

A key word I heard was 'obese', not delivered as an insult but as a defined medical term, I learned, as she explained the basic principles of BMI measurement to me. Adding to the mix, the blood pressure score was poor since despite several retakes, the numbers wouldn't improve beyond revealing me to be a Stage-2 hypertensive, one stage short of critical. Next, my blood lipid measurements, the cholesterol and triglyceride readings and the ratios between them, were all in a zone that they shouldn't be. The doctor explained the difference between the LDL (or bad) cholesterol and the good stuff (HDL), and of course I had too much of the former when compared to the latter. Finally, my blood sugars were measured as notably elevated. Again, I can't recall numbers, but I'll never forget hearing her saying the word 'pre-diabetic', which she explained was on the way to full Type 2 diabetes.

She pulled no punches with her summary: 'You are now fifty. If you don't change your ways, I don't know if you'll still be around at sixty'.

Wow. My jaw didn't literally drop to the floor, and my gob wasn't exactly smacked, but both expressions effectively summarise my immediate reaction.

I knew that my life had to change. I loved my life, I loved my wife, and I wanted to enjoy both for many, many years to follow. It was while thinking about this, and how the future could, should and would change for me, that I realised she was still talking.

The doctor explained that a number of drugs were available to help my condition, and she was able to prescribe a combination for me. But they wouldn't be effective without lifestyle changes, she said. How did I feel about that? I thought for a few seconds, and stated that I didn't fancy relying on prescribed drugs to improve my condition: 'Taking drugs all the time, that's what old and knackered people do, isn't it?', I thought in an awfully ageist way. And at some level it felt that surrendering my destiny to packets of pills was a pathetic route to take if another option was available.

So, I asked if lifestyle changes without medication could solve my issues. To my relief she said that such an approach was possible provided I was up to the challenge. Indeed, that was her preferred route for me. But it would require a substantial effort on my part, starting not next week, or tomorrow, but now. And she was talking long-term – not a month or a year but multiple years. Losing weight and increasing my health and fitness must become a priority. Diet would be key, but also exercise. Indeed, a wholesale lifestyle change would be involved.

Would I be able to do it, she wondered? So did I. After all, I'm not usually one to accept a challenge. But what I thought of next, and what I chose, would make this one of my life's most important choices, on one of the most significant days for me, ever.

I summarised the choice facing me in a three-word phrase: 'Diet or Die'.

I selected the four-letter word.

3 – Getting Started

I was ready to set the course for what would probably be the rest of my life – a life that, in my mind's eye, would be fitter, healthier and longer, and, as a result, happier.

Why 'probably'? Because this journey didn't have a known destination. Part of my employed life was as a project manager, and I felt the best way to approach this change in my life was as a project. This was definitely a project for me; the most important one I had ever undertaken. But here I was ignoring everything I had learned about goals and goal attainment. If you've heard of SMART goals, then you're ahead of me already. So, what was wrong?

- First, my goal wasn't Specific, I just wanted to lose weight and add fitness – the two high-level suggested actions from my GP. The acknowledged thinking on projects states that specific goals have a greater chance of being successful than following a general direction without a stated desired outcome. You can't score a goal if you don't know where the goalposts are. But I chose just to lose weight and add fitness.

- It wasn't Measurable, at least not directly so. Yes, the scales tell you how much you weigh, and I could probably have set myself a weight target for evaluation that way – but I didn't. I'm not sure why, probably because the GP hadn't set a goal weight. And there are many other things that could have been quantified (bodyfat percentages, blood pressure, blood sugar levels from medical measurement and perhaps speeds, distances, weights from increased activity), but again I didn't set any specific targets that would have defined success.

- Was my goal Attainable? I certainly hoped so, the warning in my GP's words had given me substantial incentive to attain it – or die through not trying. I wasn't certain I could do it – I was looking at making major changes in many aspects of my life to achieve project success. But what did success mean to me? I think I wanted something rather more from fitness than planning to visit my GP ten years' later, and saying 'Look doc, I'm still here!'. But I didn't know what that something was.

- I do of course believe that my project was Relevant, the only one of the SMART criteria that would deserve a thumbs-up. It wasn't just relevant to my life. It was critical, vital.

- Finally, I don't believe my project was Time-bound. Yes, I had the GP's ten-year number, but I didn't want fitness just to be a ten-year thing, and then check it off with a tick mark that it – whatever 'it' is – had been achieved and then move onto something else. Equally, if I had a ten-year timescale, the urge not to do anything until that deadline got closer would exist (thinking about my last-minute exam revision in years past as an example). On the other hand, if I had a metric, maybe I could have declared early victory after five years; or maybe I would find I'm not there yet after ten (but still alive to talk about it). Adding a time goal to a project is designed to make it more urgent, and prevent the project being overtaken by other priorities. I had no doubts about the importance of this project, but it's the only one I'd started that didn't have a target date or intermediate milestones on the time-line.

The project definitely needed a set of actions for me to implement, even with its ill-defined success criteria. So instead of the destination, I focussed on the journey – lose weight and become fitter. Let's not worry about how much weight and how much more fit, just go down the road to both and see how much progress I am making.

Writing those words today shocks me a little; I wouldn't settle for anything as vague as that with my personal training clients today, and many of my own fitness campaigns since that first one indeed had stated targets. But back then, losing weight and adding fitness was all I took on board. I guess it is different when you have someone working with you – such as a Personal Trainer or another member of the family. I was very much a beginner and part of me – the lazy part – was still not very enthusiastic.

It could be said that I should have sought advice at that stage. Weight loss clubs existed, and I knew where I could find a gym or two near to where we lived. I'm sure now that I could have discovered people in those places that had been where I now was, and I could learn from their experience. Why didn't I do so at the time?

At one level, I believed that I would undervalue their input as being irrelevant to me, or that they would be too demanding. I could easily envisage not following a diet regime being imposed by a nutrition expert, or being given an exercise programme from a fit person half my age which, as an obese fifty-year-old, I doubt I would achieve. Either of those would have demoralised me, perhaps sufficiently to derail the project. I'm not sure now, but perhaps I also thought they would come up with generic plans, and not take my limitations into account. More deeply, I'm not sure I wanted to own up to fitness and nutrition professionals how rubbish I had been in my eating and movement for my first fifty years that had led me to my 18 stone (252lb, 115kg) of weight.

Of course, I now realise that was a blinkered view, mixed with a level of self-esteem issues that had been brought on my perception of my body image at that time. My view was wrong. Professionals wouldn't be making such value judgements on me – nor would they have suggested nutrition or exercise plans that I couldn't accomplish. In fact, they would have congratulated me on coming to see them, highlighted this as a sign that I wanted to change, and they would have done everything to encourage me while holding me accountable to them for the results. They would have presented me with just the level of carrot and stick needed to drive me forward. Short-term goals that were SMART would have been created by them for me and my buy-in to each obtained, and they would have devised a process for each that I would feel as being within my capabilities to achieve. That's what fitness professionals do (and that's what I strive to do for my clients today).

I probably could have bought some books on nutrition and exercise, or maybe some of the magazines on these subjects. That would have been good reading on the train to and from work. But every time I looked at the magazines sold at London Bridge station on my route home, I was drawn to less demanding reading – probably something to do with railways, beer or just the Evening Standard. Also have you ever looked at the covers of fitness magazines? Not many pictures of over fifty-year-olds, nothing that drew me in. It was all far too far away from my life, far too difficult. I now recognise that was me choosing comfort eye-food, selecting easy words that I could both understand and, at a deeper level, couldn't read as being critical of my life choices so far.

So where was I now? Age fifty, obese and very unfit, and decided to embark on a major fitness project that had no specific definition of success, and chosen not to consult the very people who could have helped me make this task easier. Also, I had avoided reading anything that would provide even a generic level of guidance. Great start, Chris.

However, I was determined to reach the outcome of weighing less and becoming fitter. I didn't know at that time whether this was to be a project for the period until I considered myself changed to the required level or whether it was to be a lifestyle shift for the rest of my life. That's a big question of course, but one that didn't need an answer yet.

I knew that what I had too much of was bodyfat. That was a key thing to lose. How to go about it? I realised that bodyfat is stored fuel; and for me to be where I was at that time meant that I had over many years consumed more fuel than I'd expended in movement. What if I reversed that and started expending more than I was consuming?

I know now that there is plenty more detail around this concept, which will be covered later in this book, but unwittingly I had discovered the four most powerful words in any successful weight loss campaign:

Consume Less – Move More.

4 – A Prescription for Life: The Input

I had worked out that there were three ways I could apply that overall approach. I could move more, I could consume less, or I could do some of both.

Any of the three routes would have helped me to progress in achieving weight loss. I reasoned it was a whole lot easier doing the third option – some of both. Not just easier but probably much healthier too, as it wouldn't need such an extreme level of change in one of the variables. I decided (at last, drum roll please) to tip the balance of what is sometimes called the Energy Equation by reducing my calories inwards, and increasing my calories expended. Not a planet-shattering science discovery, but it set me on a course to follow for years ahead.

The first option is neatly summarised in the familiar old phrase 'You cannot outrun a bad diet'. And the second by a less well-known saying: 'You cannot under-eat a sedentary lifestyle'. In reality, neither of those statements are 100% true. You can indeed follow either of those approaches, but it would need extreme changes and although leaving you lighter, it certainly wouldn't make you fitter or healthier. Clearly, I would have to do route three; but by doing both actions I believed I could save going to extreme levels. I decided to move somewhat more and consume somewhat less.

Published diets were not for me. I knew, or more accurately 'suspected' since I didn't actually study any, that a standard diet would force me down routes that I wouldn't like, that wouldn't suit my lifestyle, would interfere with my social life and ban me from the foods and drinks that I enjoyed. In retrospect that probably wasn't true, but it's what I believed at the time.

I knew nothing of macronutrients, the benefits of protein, some carbs and some fats, food timing, food combination and pretty much nothing about the quality of different foods. But I did know that food and drink consumed was fuel for the body, fuel was energy and energy value was measured in calories. And it was well known that a low-calorie approach to eating and drinking could be successful. Calorie counting was my way forward. It was relatively easy, I didn't need to learn more scientific stuff (don't worry, I have now), and it is numbers-based. I like spending time playing with figures.

Things were tougher in those days for the calorie-counter. This was 2007, before every packaged food item had a nutrition label on it, and of course way before tools that can keep track of calories consumed and expended were devised. The MyFitnessPal app and the Fitbit device and their ilk were several years in the future. Thanks to those inventions life today is so much easier in terms of collecting that calories-in and calories-out data.

I purchased a couple of booklets, widely available in those days, listing calories in many of the main foods, both pre-packaged and raw materials. I bought two as I soon discovered each booklet covered different food groups in more detail. Either would have given me about 80% of the data, put the two together and I made it about 90% with massive overlap, which would do. You won't see them in magazine shops these days as all this information is now available online.

Using the information from the booklets and adding my own estimates for the 10% of items I ate that weren't listed in either of the books, I reckoned I was eating somewhere between 3000 and 3500 calories on a typical day, 50% more than I probably should have been consuming. Just typing those numbers today sends a shiver through my system.

I set myself a new figure of 1600 calories as the daily target input I would aim at – at least initially. Where did I derive this number from? I don't know – maybe I read it, maybe I invented it. It is about 50% of the level I was eating before, and that seemed about right. So, 1600 calories it was. I still didn't know any of the other variables which affect the transformation of food consumed into bodyfat, but I had a number to work with. That 1600 number was the most unscientifically arrived-at number around, but it was there. I carved it in virtual stone and it became a significant part of my life for many months to follow.

I couldn't have followed a health-food only diet. I wanted to lose weight, not lose enjoyment from life. This was a key factor for me, and is key for success in any weight loss regime. Maybe I should patent it: 'The Chris Zaremba Enjoyable Diet' – C-ZED would have been a nice acronym.

Mindset is very important if goals are going to be achieved and a miserable Chris wasn't what I was after. I decided that, whatever I did, I wasn't going to be a misery to myself or others and I would still very much enjoy a beer or meal out with friends. Saying to Shawn or Richard: 'Sorry, I can't come out for a beer tonight because I can't afford the calories' just wasn't going to happen. Something less rigid was needed but it still had to work within that 1600 number.

My approach was to eat and drink less overall, keeping everything I enjoyed but at a reduced volume, and make sensible substitutions wherever possible. To keep track of my progress I purchased a little spiral bound notebook to record each day, a page per day. On that page, I listed what I ate – a brief description then the calories of that item alongside and the total-so-far today on the right. Initially, I only did the summation at the end of each day, but of course that didn't help in managing the rest of any day after the initial meals; so that cumulative column went in from about day three.

I set myself three special rules:

- Meals out with Jenny and friends, or on business, all count as 1000 calories. These meals are the hardest to calorie count. Also, I didn't want to spend time that I should be enjoying the company of my dining companions by thinking of calories and getting my little notebook out. Any meal out counted as 1000 calories, whatever it is, provided it's without bread and dessert (fruit allowed) and with any alcohol to be added as extra on top of the 1000.

- Carry-forward is allowed. Any allowance unused from one day could be carried forward to the next; equally, any deficit too. So, if I ended up with 2000 calories consumed on one day – with nothing having been brought forward – then I carried -400 forward to the next day, giving me just 1200 for that next day. To even it out, I would probably have gone for around 1400 that second day, with a -200 carried forward to the third day. All recorded in the notebook, of course.

- Estimate. The numbers in calorie guides are themselves estimates of values. A level of daily precision that I believed was correct to the nearest 100 at the end of the day did it for me. But I counted everything, even if I couldn't find a value from my books. An estimated value is far better than an ignored value.

One tip that I learned after a couple of weeks was the immense value in planning. I've much more to say about this later, but this was when I first learned how much the planning of a day could help to achieve my goals. If I knew what I was going to be doing that evening and could plan the estimated calories for it, I could adjust to consume fewer during the day. I moved to writing the notebook page on the train to London every morning with my list of what I was planning to consume that day, the calories and, as a new first column, at what time. Writing this also provided something for my hands to do now that I didn't have the on-train Mars Bar to eat. I had a guide to follow for that day and I regarded it as a victory if I followed it. And if anything unexpected came up, I could delete what I had written and replan the rest of the day.

When I was tempted by something, I performed an evaluation. How many calories is it? Is it worth that number of calories from the daily target? How does that affect the plan for what I can eat for the rest of the day? If I performed this test and it yielded positive answers, then I went for it. This sounds a laborious process but it wasn't. I applied this test multiple times a day and very soon it was virtually instantaneous.

I started devising ways to keep my enjoyment up while reducing calories. It took me a few weeks, but I learned to like tea and coffee without sugar. A few weeks later, and I starting taking them without milk as well. That reduced calories per cup from 100 to zero. I had also taken a liking to cappuccino coffee, which can be upwards of 150. Three cappuccinos replaced by black coffee? That's 400 or more calories saved! That was a big, relatively easy win.

Main meals weren't much different to before, but fish and chips comes in at 800 – wow. That's a special treat and not as it had been, sometimes a near-daily occurrence, often as a prelude to dinner. I deduced that main courses at lunch and dinner didn't have to change too much, but the snacks and nibbles in between were a regular source of calories that I could live without.

I stopped putting sugar on cereals and moved to skimmed milk, and switched to low-calorie versions of everything. Generally speaking, desserts were out, as were cakes and biscuits, and bread with a restaurant meal. I had developed a taste for the fine, sophisticated and subtle flavour of a Big Mac meal, but discovered that the calories were halved if I missed out the fries (of which I didn't actually enjoy the taste anyway) and if I took the diet drink.

And other things that I particularly liked were possible, but not in large portions and not daily. As you have read, I was, and still am, a big supporter of traditional real ale, which averages about 200 calories a pint. So, I could have two a day, and still have 1200 remainder: not bad. I could have two pints and still have 1400 left if I carried forward the shortfall, or better still, utilise the -200 today that I'd brought forward from yesterday just for such an occasion - the value of planning indeed.

I'm beginning to sound like an alcoholic, which I wasn't (at least, I don't think so). I realised that a bottle of beer, drunk with small sips from the bottle, was the social and duration equivalent of a pint but with half the calories; a good way of saving some extra calories there, and helping my liver as a side-benefit. Crisps and salted peanuts do not in themselves bring much joy, but were a habit for me as for many, one that people don't think about that much. (Brewers do – the salt makes you want to drink more), so often a few packets are added on to a round of drinks. After some thought I skipped those too and that's another 150 or so calories saved.

On my daily routine, the chocs had to go. Sorry to Cadbury and Mars, but the three or more of your products I had daily were taking up maybe 700 of my precious calories. When I did want to munch on something, so I took to an apple or other fruit instead, but not as often, since there were more shops selling chocs than fruit on my regular travels for these ad-hoc purchases.

I should have had enough inputs to motivate, inspire and encourage me to be immediately successful on this new approach to eating. All the information I needed was there. I just needed to follow my rules and live by them. It doesn't sound easy, and to start with it wasn't. Even though I massively wanted to change, my willpower wasn't up to putting all the elements of the new nutrition approach into place at one go. As is so often the case in matters related to fitness, small steps often lead to major achievements, providing you keep taking the small steps.

I found that by changing just one thing at a time, seeing how I managed with that, then another thing, and so on, worked for me and led in time to a complete diet overhaul. My willpower also coped better with making small changes at intervals rather than attempting any major change. As a result, the transition from my old way of eating to the new way took around a year, during which time I gradually dropped the nasty old habits and incorporated new healthy eating strategies.

Often, I found that these small steps led one to another in a linked way – usually two, three or even more steps to replace one bad eating habit with a good one. For example, I initially replaced my cereals with more natural products such as Alpen with milk as first stage, then Sugar-Free Alpen as a second, then making porridge from rolled oats, then finally swapping the milk for water with the oats.

Another example was cutting down take-aways from around five per week initially to twice a week then on to only rarely. A third example was moving the soft drink of choice from full-sugar Coke to Diet Coke initially, then as a further stage on to bottled water. Even for small things, there were multi-stage changes: coffee at home with milk and two sugars became coffee with skimmed milk and one sugar, then black coffee on its own.

Frequently for these types of change, I had no idea a second or third stage was waiting when I made the initial shift. The subsequent step presented itself in time as the next thing to alter once I had achieved my first level change on one aspect and wanted to progress further from that point. There was never a master plan of the intermediate steps in getting to new nutrition principles. I knew where I started from and I more or less knew where I wanted to end up, but the process of reaching the end position was a gradual process of those small steps, each of which was made up as I progressed. I doubt I would have been successful had I approached it in any other way.

It probably would have been so much easier with a huge dollop of willpower. I didn't think I had much, but I found that the death sentence from my GP was a remarkable motivator, one I thought about most days. The willpower had a massive level of ingrained behaviour to overcome. My eating and drinking habits had been developing for fifty years and they weren't going away without a fight. Over time, as those small steps eventually took me down a healthier path, the neural pathways were redrawn and the brain and hormones became used to different tastes and expectations of volume. And that's exactly what happened, and that's how I made 1600 calories a day work for me for the next two years.

But I'm getting ahead of myself here. I've only looked at one half of the Energy Equation so far and in parallel with this reduction of input, my self-prescribed route needed an increase in output.

5 – A Prescription for Life: The Output

It is hard to convey how inactive I was in those days before receiving the warning from my GP. I wasn't exaggerating in Chapter 1 when I said how games and PE were unhappy times at school. I didn't enjoy exercise then, and that did not change in the decades that followed. Playing squash was an exception to this but that stopped when my Achilles Tendon gave way, as I've explained. I found that my Achilles held up for a few steps of running, but I don't believe I ran more than ten metres in one go from that date until the day of my GP's warning. And to be honest I wouldn't have run those ten metres unless I really was desperate to catch that bus or heard 'last orders' in the distance.

It is true to say that I had a shock coming to my body. I knew I couldn't run, not significantly so anyway, but I also knew I had to increase my energy output. You know that I like numbers and counting calories on food was fine for that. I couldn't work out a way of similarly quantifying my energy spent (I can now) but I knew that something was better than nothing, so it was back to the standard ill-defined success criteria.

One thing I learned early on is that it is movement we are talking about here, not specifically exercise. Setting aside a specific time for it and (heaven forbid!) going to a gym was not required. But it was movement itself that counted and the more movement the better, I reasoned to myself.

To start off with I wasn't up to allocating specific times in my daily life for this extra activity that I wanted to incorporate in to my daily life. As you know, I was commuting to London by train in those days and I found that I could make changes in my routine that would enable me to find some additional movement in my life, but minimising adding time for exercise. At the time, I lived around fifteen minutes' walk from the local station, Cheam, and had a fifteen-minute walk at the other end, from London Bridge to my office. I reckon I walked maybe half of the trips at the home end and caught a bus or a lift on the other half. And at the London end it was always a tube or bus both ways. On average my usual behaviour had been to walk one out of four or those daily commuting legs.

This was the first stop on the route to improvement. I found an average of an extra 45 minutes walking a day by eliminating those three times as a passenger. I found as the days passed that it wasn't taking me much longer to walk than to use transport. Queuing for the bus (as we did in those days) and slow traffic actually meant that each leg as a passenger probably cost me ten minutes anyway. Even when the weather turned for the worse, I managed to keep walking as this was no longer a journey to work but part of my quest to lose weight. I was walking to work and getting fitter in the same period of time. This ability to hit two objectives from one time period was key to me in finding time for exercise and it is something I stress to my clients to this day – finding ways to benefit from lots of added exercise for little added time.

I know friends who have taken up walking and they buy audio books or listen to podcasts to make the walk more enjoyable. In those days audio books or podcasts hadn't been invented. The voice in my head was me, telling me to keep going, remembering why I was doing this, and that mental focus worked.

Looking back, making those changes into four fifteen-minute walks rather than rides was a win on so many fronts – lots of added exercise for little added time, the health and weight-loss benefits of using muscles to power and fat to fuel the trip, improved mental health from not worrying about traffic delays and in case the bus were to be full, some slightly fresher air than inside the vehicle (this was London, not the Lake District, I can't claim it really was fresh air); and I saved myself the cost of the fare. So apart from the increased wear on my shoes, where was the downside in any of that?

I worked on the fourth floor of an office building then, and another easy win was to set a personal policy of always walking up and down the stairs rather than using the lifts. And often I had to go to visit another office on the eighth floor and adopted the same policy, using the stairs from fourth to eighth and back again. With going out at lunchtime, I reckon I was climbing up twelve storeys of the building each working day. And again, I don't think it took too much extra time. Yes, the lifts travelled faster than I climbed, but factoring in the wait time I think I probably broke even on timing. I've just realised that I had mentally set four permanently as my number for storeys climbed and I still use that as a guideline measure today. In any office building I still default to taking a lift if there are five or more floors to ascend and walk if it is less.

I added a few other policies to cover most of the rest of the day. I would go for a walk at lunchtime if there wasn't a team drink taking place, walk up escalators when I was on the tube, and so on. Basically, I was looking for opportunities to get some movement in without having to allocate additional time for it. On an average office day, I was probably walking 5km more than before as well as climbing those twelve storeys, both without much extra time.

After about two weeks of this I decided to up my game. I joined a gym, located next to my office. The membership fee was about the same as three pints of beer a week and my beer consumption was down by at least that amount. Those savings alone easily covered gym costs. I remember specifically not telling any of my beer friends about joining. They would have poured scorn on it as quickly as they poured ale down their throats and that wouldn't have helped me mentally. I wasn't anywhere near certain that gym membership would suit me, or that I wouldn't always find excuses not to go. But I regularly recalled that doctor's warning about increasing my fitness levels. I was internally conflicted and I avoided adding external conflict to that by not telling my friends. This was a big mistake, as I found out later.

Back to the gym: I reasoned that it was easy to visit during lunchtime at the office. You now know what I'm like and I didn't take any advice. I probably had a gym induction session, but if I did, I don't remember it now and didn't remember anything I was told back then.

Ears were closed, but eyes were open. I saw the weights area with guys who appeared to know what they were doing. None of them looked like they needed to be in a gym, certainly not compared to me. I instantly felt insecure, doubly obese and massively over-age for this place. I didn't belong here. All of these people working out were way fitter than I ever wanted to be anyway, and yet they were still here, still feeling the need to improve. I would stick out like at least an obese-sized sore thumb here; and even if I lost the weight and became super-fit, I'd still be old enough to be the father of any of them, and still wouldn't belong here. Definitely, avoid all of this. Anyway, what does lifting weights do? Builds muscle, right? Muscle weighs something, yes? I wanted to lose weight, not gain it. I persuaded myself that wasn't the area for me and yielded to my perceived inadequacies.

The next thing I remember seeing was the group exercise studio. There was a class in progress at the time. They were mainly women, all half my age or less and already way more than twice my fitness on average. Most of them were moving and not sweating as far as I could see. This was even more of a no-no for me than the weights area. I knew I would be useless at anything I was asked to do, since I hadn't moved that much in decades, in fact probably ever. I thought that everyone else in the class would laugh at this older, fatter, sweaty, inept bloke pretending he had a right to be here. And if any activity involved breaking the group up into sections for a race (it probably wouldn't, but I was assuming the worst), then I would undoubtedly be last and holding my section up. So, you can add my team-sport inadequacies to the self-esteem problems I've described earlier. As I've mentioned already, some of those insecurities still exist to some level in me. I don't like group exercise classes to this day, even though I'm qualified to teach some of them; and I still retain my team-member peer pressure issues as a hangover from school.

I was beginning to feel that I had made a huge mistake somewhere. I didn't want to be a fitness enthusiast like everyone I saw in the gym. I was only here because my doctor ordered me to lose weight. Glumness abounded. However (you knew this had to happen eventually) things changed for the positive. I saw the cardiovascular training area, and gradually my spirits perked up. Here there was no concept of doing anything as a group or as a team or in any form of race. There was no one to study my performance, as everyone was watching screens or the displays on their machines, maybe listening to headsets, all facing forwards, so no one would be watching me. Most of the machines had displays of numbers, which are a dispassionate and objective presentation of what was being achieved, not human beings forming opinions and involved in a subjective assessment of my performance.

Some of the people taking part even looked a bit like me, the first people I had seen in the place who actually appeared to need a bit of gym work. I would no doubt sweat, but they were doing so too, and unashamedly so. This had a chance of working. I could see myself doing stuff here.

What should have been next was to speak to one of the trainers there for advice on choosing the cardio equipment to use. However, my lack of confidence at the time and silly belief that no one would take an obese bloke of over fifty seriously in the gym won in my head, so it was all experimentation without guidance.

I tried out all the cardio equipment the next day at a time when there weren't many people around. I decided that each item of kit had advantages and disadvantages in its use, particularly as applied to me as a fifty-year old with a very unfit body. Mostly my evaluation of their worth and relevance to my fitness situation were made rapidly and more on gut-feel than evidence; but even without advice at the time I think my assessments weren't far off.

Firstly, I decided that running on the treadmill and climbing the Stairmaster (a continuously rotating conveyor belt of steps to climb, forever upwards) were both too hard. I would come to love the treadmill in time, but not yet. I could have set the treadmill to walk, I suppose. But, hang on, I was walking at lunchtime anyway out on the streets and lots to and from work, so it didn't really seem to offer anything extra, while taking time for changing. And why pay to walk when I could do that for nothing?

The rowing machine made my lower back hurt and I found the stationary bike just a bit too easy and not giving enough return for my time, probably because the body is supported and stationary. I reasoned (correctly as it happens) that I wouldn't derive the most energy-used-per-minute from it compared to other cardio options due to sitting down all the time. Remember I had a lot of kilos to be used as deadweight in any cardio exercise and being seated wouldn't use that bulk to my calorie-burning advantage.

At last, I found the cross-trainer (or elliptical trainer). Having dismissed most of the options offered in cardio equipment, here was something I could relate to. It used my serious bodyweight as a resistance, was more effort than walking (good), but wasn't as much effort as running (very good). I had worked out that more effort means more calories burned, and I had now found something that would use more energy per minute than my lunchtime walks, and yet not so hard that I would stop after a very few minutes.

Was I overjoyed to find it? No. I still didn't want to be here. I was only doing this as part payment of the debt I owed to my body after years of treating it badly. If I hadn't made that visit to my GP and if my flying licence had still been valid, then I would have been happy never to enter this building. Yet I knew I had to make the best of my situation, and in the cross-trainer, I had found something which I could do that I wouldn't hate, and that would help me in following that doctor's prescription.

I started going every lunchtime. I found I could change clothes, do twenty minutes exercise, have a quick shower, buy a sandwich within my daily calorie plan and be back at my desk all within my lunch hour. I quickly extended that by twenty minutes to double the exercise time, which made me twenty minutes late back from lunch. I found that extra twenty minutes by going at 11:50, which I mentally rounded up to 12:00, and coming back at 1:10 (rounded down to 1:00). I hoped my boss used the same rounding algorithm.

This timing wasn't ideal. I didn't know how long I would get away with sneaking those extra twenty minutes, and I didn't want to miss out on lunchtime drinks (calorie-counted, of course) with friends and colleagues. In fact, I didn't miss out. I went to nearly all of them. I probably only actually hit the cross-trainer on 50% of my office days. I wanted to lose weight, not enjoyment or friends, so something had to change. But I needed the to burn the calories somehow.

What changed was my timing. I switched the cardio to before work. I could cope with the forty-minutes timing on the cross-trainer and didn't want to cut down, so I devised a new policy of getting to the gym at 8:00, cross-trainer then shower, pick up breakfast, take to office and eat at my desk. And I made my desk by about 9:10 (which, as you now know, rounds down to 9:00). This saved a little time as I didn't do all my pre-work tasks at home. I showered after my cardio not after waking and I tied my tie (it was that long ago, we wore ties) before leaving the gym, not before leaving home. I found that I could do 40 minutes of pre-office cardio plus a shower by getting up only 50 minutes earlier; and I was still doing the two walks between home and the station, and from my London terminus to the gym then to the office every morning.

My prescription was complete and I was able to follow it. I was getting into a daily routine, a habit. It didn't need much conscious effort to adhere to it. How did I feel? Tired and hungry, as my calorie consumption dropped and my calorie usage grew. I weighed myself at the gym. I can't remember the exact numbers for these early months in my fitness life, but I can remember a noticeable drop in my weight.

That, of course, made me feel good because I was at last making some headway. I wasn't enjoying it, but I was putting in the hard labour that my doctor had judged that my condition justified.

Something very significant happened after a couple of months. I had to go to a business meeting in Leeds and had to travel on an early train. I found myself trying to work out whether I could find time to do the cardio first before heading to King's Cross. I even thought about how I could squeeze it in on my return to London that evening, if I took my gym clothes to Yorkshire with me. I worked out that, sadly, I couldn't.

Stop! Look at that last sentence again. Particularly the third word from the end.

I was actually regretting not having time to do the cardio. What had happened is that somehow, miraculously, this extra exercise I was doing had turned into something I enjoyed doing, rather than something I was doing reluctantly as a result of the doctor's orders. I realised that I wasn't doing the cardio, nor the extra walks and stairs, not even the calorie-restricted input, because I had to. I was doing these things because I wanted to. That change had probably been creeping up on me ever since I had started the fitness project and signed up to my gym routine, but I didn't realise it until that very moment.

I call it my Magic Moment. It was life-changing.

6 – On the Right Track, Almost

From that moment to this I have never felt that I was doing any kind of exercise at the request or order of someone else. I'm not saying I've always gone to every one of my planned exercise sessions, nor that I actually enjoyed them all, but my decision to go or not to go was my own. I could do what I wanted, and usually that meant rising early and doing some exercise. But I never felt that I was letting anyone down if I didn't do it. I had definitely turned my thoughts away from following my GP's recommendation. My 'inner voice' was providing all the inspiration that I needed.

We are now about the middle of 2007. Around three months since I was with the GP, three months during which I'd set myself on a course of calories in going down, and calories out going up. The plan for the future was very simple: more of the same, until…. well, I didn't really know until when, but let's keep going because (a) I am enjoying it, (b) I am sure my GP would approve and (c) Jenny thought it a very good use of my time.

It's time for a few paragraphs on the detail of my cardio on the cross-trainer. If you're not familiar with the breed, let me introduce you. It's a machine where you run with feet on individual footplates that move, powered by you, in an elliptical motion by alternately pushing down on one side while being supported on the other. There are handles to use for extra movement, should you want to use them. Resistance can be varied if required. Simply put, it's an easier form of running, much lower-impact, but with a good rate of calorie burn, depending of course on the combination of speed you go and the resistance level you set. Every gym has a number of them in their cardio area.

The cross-trainer had become a substantial part of my daily life by that stage and I wanted to use it to optimum effect. I read somewhere (possibly on a cross-trainer notice or a gym wall poster) about heart rate zones and noted that maximum fat burn was said to occur between 70% and 80% of maximum heart rate, with that maximum being calculated as 220 minus age. I now know there is a whole load more detail attached to that but at the time that was enough science for me. I had purchased a heart rate monitor (and indeed many cross-trainers have that functionality built in) so (hooray) I could now start playing with numbers.

Those percentages gave me a heart rate target of between 110 and 144 beats per minute (bpm). The mid-point of that is 127 and I set that as my target. Obviously, it takes a few minutes to reach that level but the majority of the forty minutes was at or near that point. I controlled the heart rate by a combination of the level of resistance and speed. I enjoyed then (still do, actually) playing with those two variables to produce the bpm I want. I invested in one of the early model iPod Shuffles, loaded some of my favourite tracks on it and used the beat of the music to govern my speed. I found it far easier to Jump To The Beat than not, so I was truly in a Boogie Wonderland on that cross-trainer. You are beginning to spot my iPod playlist, and, having started, Don't Stop Me Now. Yes, I agree. I will stop that now.

There are three variables to play with that affect the heart rate: time, resistance level and speed. Time wasn't a factor. I'd settled on forty minutes being the duration and I never varied, so this was not much of a variable in my case. As I don't change my pace mid-music track, any change in my heart rate has to come from adjustments in the resistance level. To save constantly checking if I was on target, I checked only once per minute and made the adjustment to the level at that point. As it's almost impossible to keep a fixed bpm and since I didn't want to change every single minute, I set myself a target range for cardio of 125-130 bpm. The rule I applied was: check on the minute, if my heart rate is below the target range, move the resistance level up one; and if my rate is above, then move it down one. I found that starting at a resistance level of 12 on that particular model and following that rule meant that most of my cardio was at a level of 16, which suited me well.

I read up a little about it – yes actually doing some research for a change – and found the additional cross-trainer benefits of being low-impact on the joints and using the arms. The low-impact comes from the footplates travelling with your feet and supporting them at all points of the movement. Using the arms of the machine provides a bit of a workout for the upper body, and moving the arms also counts as calorie-burning movement of course. If this is reading as if I knew what I was talking about, then – yes, it's true, I had learned of the benefits of the cross-trainer and was very keen to continue to use the machine as a key part of my weight loss programme.

Nothing fundamental happened to change my fitness project for over a year. There is one more gobsmacking, fundamental moment still to come, the third if you are counting, but you'll have to wait until the end of 2008 for that. That will not actually be too long in this narrative.

What had started out as being doctor's orders had become a pleasure, and was now a way of life that I could mould to fit everything else I was doing. I had to miss my weekday morning cardio often due to business meetings and on those occasions, I would try to fit it in later in the day. That wasn't always possible, but usually I could find a spot with some planning the night before. My gym was one of the national chains, Cannons, and I upgraded my membership so that I could use their gyms in other locations if that made sense when business trips disrupted my gym trips. I was still getting away with my rounding errors on timing at the office, and I found that taking an unusually long time to come back from a visit to a client was ideal for sneaking in my day's cardio. And renting a permanent locker at the gym next to the office meant I wasn't spotted carrying gym kit when I left for that business meeting, or bringing it back. I was being a bit creative, juggling times to drop kit off, doing the cardio and picking it up later. The last time I was regularly this sneaky was when I was trying to avoid doing exercise at school, now I was using the same level of deviousness to do the exact opposite. It's a funny old world sometimes.

There was a Cannons gym fifteen minutes from our house so I used my multi-club access to make sure that I could fit my cardio sessions in at the weekend as well. I was hooked on the cross-trainer daily, or as near daily as possible. I think I missed my cardio no more than once or twice per month throughout that first eighteen months. I coupled that with what I had learned about energy in everyday activity: walking when possible, and ideally walking quickly, taking the stairs rather than lift, walking up escalators. I was always looking for means to burn extra calories in life without allocating any gym time in addition to my cardio to do it.

I've mentioned that Jenny is a keen triathlete, and she was pleased to see the progress I was making. She wanted to ensure that we shouldn't be spending too much time apart during my fitness campaign so I promised her that when I was fit enough, I'd join her on some of her bike rides. And as winter turned to spring that indeed happened, as you'll read about in more detail in Chapter 21. We did cycle rides together to a level of fitness that was still basic for Jenny but was definitely a substantial upgrade for me. She encouraged me (mainly by the ploy of routing our bike rides to end at good pubs) and was happy to know that my cycling would now come with less likelihood of imminent cardiac arrest.

Talking of pubs takes me back to the first half of the Energy Equation, the input. I was still using the small notebook at this point to record calories-in. I was tempted to drop that since I was beginning to have a good feel for what would be a good day's eating without writing it down. But I decided to keep the system going. With hindsight, that was the right decision. 'What gets written, gets done' is one of my favourite sayings in fitness.

It was of major importance to me that I maintained my joy in life outside of fitness. I don't think I ever rejected a night out, a beer or two, or the occasional pub-crawl with Jenny and/or my beery chums. I wasn't in this fitness project to become miserable, as I've mentioned before. But I did notice my tastes change over these months. I found that full-sugar soft drinks had become sickly sweet to my taste buds, along with anything with added sugar. Did I really put sugar on Shredded Wheat or Weetabix? I'm not going to claim that I cut down substantially on my beloved traditional real ale but I continued to eliminate the things that went with it – the crisps, nuts, then the pasty, kebab van, burger or fish and chips on the way home. But this was not only because of the calories, but also because my tastes were changing. I didn't make the decision to ban anything. Many items banned themselves as I just didn't fancy them anymore. Even chocolate, to which I was probably addicted, started to have a fatty and oversweet mouth feel to it, and I just became fed up with it after a relatively small amount. Up to that point I didn't know that it was possible to eat just a couple of chocolate digestives because I used to wolf down most of the packet at one sitting.

I wish I could tell you how many calories I was taking in and expending at this time. It would make a really powerful statement at this point in the narrative to say 'I used to consume x calories and expend y, but those figures had become...' But I can't. In these days before technology came to my help, the only number that sticks in my head is that forty minutes on the cross-trainer, according to the machine, burned around 400 calories of energy. However, I knew that this was just for an average person, based on speed, resistance and duration of the exercise, but didn't take into account resting, the user's heart rate, weight, age and several other variables that would be needed for an accurate number specific to one person.

So, here am I, a numbers-geek, unable to give you even basic numbers for my energy consumed and used for this period. I could of course refer to that notebook recording calories taken in, had I not lost it years ago (all three volumes of it by that stage). However, I'm sure it is accurate to say that x in that last paragraph used to be substantially more than y, now it was the other way round.

I did keep a basic track of my weight. I used the scales in the gym and put a daily value on that day's page in my calorie-record notebook. At that point, around 18 months after my doctor's warning, I recall having come down from 18 stone to 15 stone (252lb to 210lb, 114kg to 95kg). That works out to around 0.5lb per week, or 1kg per month. I am not going to claim that's the best rate of weight loss around, but it was sustainable for me for that period and it allowed me to eat pretty much what I wanted to by that time. I remember adjusting my calories-in target at some point to 2000 a day with the same carry-forward system as before, and I would no doubt have had a quicker rate of loss to show if I'd stuck to 1600. But I wasn't on a diet and I hated the word. It had such negative connotations for me. Instead, I was eating in accordance with my lifestyle, a weight-loss lifestyle where I enjoyed most food and drink in reasonable quantities most of the time.

So, I definitely thought everything was going well. I had lost three stone, what could possibly be going wrong? But I had made an error in my fitness life. A major mistake. Have you spotted it?

I discovered it in September 2008, while on holiday nearly 6000 miles from home.

7 – The Next Revelation

I had no idea that something was wrong. I had lost around forty pounds in weight in eighteen months, I had eased up on my lowered calorie input figure but I was still losing weight. Most of all, I was enjoying it – both the exercise and the nutrition approach that gave me the freedom to eat what I wanted, in sensible amounts, and still continue with the weight loss. I could easily envisage carrying on that way; if I continued at the same rate, which was entirely possible as I had found this approach to be sustainable, in three years I would have lost six stone. Which would take me down to twelve stone (168lb, 76kg), and that would make me a happy chappy indeed.

As I said, I had no idea that something was going wrong. But it was – very wrong.

It was late 2008, I was 51 and on holiday in Santa Monica, California. 'On holiday' is perhaps stretching it a bit, Jenny had a reason to be there on business for a week; I decided to take a week off work and join her. Not quite gate-crashing her trip, but certainly sharing the hotel room which she would have used anyway. Jenny and I agreed that, of course, I would keep out of her way while she was working – that was every weekday and indeed most evenings.

Keeping out of the way meant four things to occupy myself – (1) trying out the local interesting beers, as the microbrewery explosion in the USA was just starting, (2) going for a few day-trip train rides – such as to San Diego and Santa Barbara, (3) taking some flying lessons, just for familiarity with the procedures as I still wanted to keep my hand in while being medically disqualified from flying, and of course (4) my daily gym cardio. It's this fourth point where the plot thickens.

Our hotel, correction, Jenny's hotel, didn't have a gym and I wanted to find one to buy a week's membership for my daily cross-training. Gyms aren't exactly scarce in Southern California, but I knew the most famous nearby was called Gold's – so I found it and took a week's membership.

It's a huge place, easily ten times the size of any other gym I'd been in. And masses of equipment, three rooms – hangars would be a more accurate term – with just about every usable square foot occupied by free weights, resistance machines, and devotees working with them. And a relatively small cardiovascular training area. This was a gym where cardio definitely came second to muscle-building. I was amazed by some of the clientele – trying hard not to stare, many of these guys were huge, with muscles in places where I didn't even have places. It seemed unnatural that some of these gym-goers could be so large, so muscled and still be the same species as me (I later learned that, for many of them, nature had little to do with it).

I was awed, but not intimidated or jealous. I would have been massively intimidated eighteen months earlier, but my daily gym visits had removed those insecurities for the most part. I knew I was allowed to be in this place – well, maybe not the weights rooms, but in the cardio area at least. And I absolutely wasn't jealous; as I've said before, I had decided that muscle weighs, and my project was about reducing my bodyweight, not increasing it. That was reason enough, but to add to that, I didn't like the bodybuilder look – the proportions seemed all wrong, was it really healthy and doesn't it take the dedication of training all day, every day to look like that? Nope, each to their own, but that's not for me; I would leave the weights to the big boys, I was content to stay in that cardiovascular area.

I said that the cardio area was a relatively small proportion of the floor space at Gold's. But it was still far bigger in actual terms than in any other gym I had visited. Probably around 100 machines – all the usual ones, plus a handful new to me. I tried one of the new ones – the Jacob's Ladder, which is a conveyor belt angled upwards at around 20 degrees to the horizontal, with rungs that can be used for feet and

47

hands to constantly climb, but without actually ascending anywhere. Rather like the endless climb of a Stairmaster but with hands involved. I could see it would be a big calorie burner, but I didn't like looking downwards all the time and I couldn't easily do in synch with my iPod music. So, I stuck to the familiar cross-trainer, every morning for the usual 40 minutes. In summary, I had come thousands of miles, joined the world's most famous and well-equipped gym, and was doing... exactly what I did at home. One view: you stick-in-the-mud, Chris. Another view: why change a winning formula?

On day four, I finally discovered what was wrong. Let's slip back to day three first; the weather forecast was for rain all day tomorrow (yes, it does sometimes rain in Southern California), therefore no flying training was likely to happen and, thanks to the rain, I didn't want to do a soggy day riding the rails to somewhere new, even with some interesting beer at the destination. I would therefore have extra time on my hands. I'd noticed a sign near the Reception area of Gold's promoting personal training. A bit of me said, well, I know I'll never be a regular with weights, but I might as well give that a go. I had no idea what really was involved, but with loads of spare time, if not now, when? And if not here, where? I asked the receptionist, he gave me the contact details of a personal trainer he knew called Rob Riches, and advised me to send him an email. 'You'll like Rob, he's just like you', he added.

Rob and I agreed to meet at Gold's the next day. The receptionist had been wrong. He wasn't just like me. Not even a bit, really. True, he wasn't one of the massive bodybuilders that I'd taken an aversion to back on Gold's day one, but he was certainly well-muscled, and didn't look like he carried anything that could be called bodyfat. He radiated health and fitness. And I guessed he was well under half my age. 'Just like me'. Really? I couldn't spot the similarity from looking. Then I found out the what we had in common that gave the receptionist that view – Rob spoke with the same accent as me, London-area English.

I had booked an hour personal training session with Rob, but was a little nervous – I didn't know what to expect. I'd never had any gym personal training of any sort, what I wanted (I thought) was for someone to show me a few interesting exercises with weights, and that's what I told Rob I wanted to do – but he decided he needed to know more about me first. We sat in the small part of the gym area devoted to conversation, and we talked about my story. At some length, covering everything relevant from Chapter 2 of this book right up to that day, and my plan of continuing on my successful weight-loss journey for another eighteen months to make it a full six stone lost. Nice to be talking, of course, but I was actually beginning to think that we weren't going to touch a weight in that hour.

Rob asked many questions – a couple I remember is 'Why no weight training so far?' – he gently smirked at my answer that I didn't want to put on muscle as I was trying to lose weight. I thought that was the correct answer; his little laugh had told me otherwise. And he sought confirmation on my nutrition – 'You're not keeping your protein intake up?' – I replied that I didn't do that level of analysis on my food, I liked to keep to my calorie target but I had no idea how much was protein. 'But it is all good, Rob, I've lost forty pounds in weight!'

I was beginning to feel I was being told off, or – more accurately – being made to make myself realise that I'd missed something massive here. Then Rob came back with the killer paragraph, which I am trying to remember as accurately as possible – 'It's really great that you've lost that weight, Chris, but a lot of what you have lost is muscle. You're getting lighter, yes, but less fit and definitely weaker. Carry on what you are doing for another eighteen months as you say and you will have changed into a scrawny weakling. The body naturally loses muscle at your age; you are accelerating that process with your fitness project'.

I'm not sure he actually used the term 'scrawny weakling', but the definition of scrawny is 'unattractively thin and bony', and that is what he meant.

Oh, sugar! And I thought I was doing so well, too.

8 – Resistance isn't Useless

And this was my introduction to weight training. The logic that Rob had used in reaching his conclusion on me made perfect sense; I was losing weight, but that loss had been accomplished by a reduction in muscle mass as well as loss of some bodyfat. I hadn't lost any muscles, of course, but the mass of each of my muscles had been reduced – less mass, less size, less strength. Mass is weight, so some of my weight loss had been that muscle mass.

I knew then my mission had to make a fundamental change – Rob told me, but I had already worked out, that I needed to add back the muscle that my previous months of weight loss had taken away.

But I didn't want to add overall weight. I was now down to 15 stone (210lb, 95kg) and I knew I could and should go further. I wanted to add back the muscle mass – and, as I've mentioned before, muscle weighs, right? So, what I wanted was to know how to reset my activities such that I could both lose bodyfat as I had been doing, but now add back muscle.

I asked Rob how to continue to lose bodyfat, but add muscle mass. Little did I realise it back then, but that is the ultimate question in any form of weight training or fitness activity – whether international standard bodybuilder or weekend runner. It's a question that does have answers – not just an answer, I found that many differing views exist on the best approach to accomplish that. Rob told me his views – but not until the following day. I'll keep you waiting too – not until tomorrow, just a few chapters.

Rob had to go back to some basic anatomy, including a trick question – he asked if I knew how many biceps I had. Fairly sure on that, two. So how many triceps, Chris? I went for three. And did I know the difference between dumbbells and barbells? Not sure on that one. I knew that it wasn't to do with the first being quieter than the second, or the second being the tab at my local, but that was about it. As we headed to the first exercise, Rob knew he had his work cut out.

I can't remember now which exercises he showed me, but for each he explained how it should be performed safely and to good effect, then gave a demo, then I had a go and did something wrong. I learned that patience and empathy are just two of the qualities in a good personal trainer – one that I hope I have when training my own clients today.

Each of the three massive gym rooms at Gold's was laid out with benches, weights on racks and mirrors everywhere. I was particularly intrigued by the large and complex machines, all levers, cables and pulleys – plus somewhere to sit while the machine does its worst on you. Judging by some of the grunting and groaning going on around me, these were different sorts of self-inflicted torture devices. But looking closely for the first time, I became fascinated by each; how does this one work, Rob, and can I have a go now? I had a well-qualified guide to this particular chamber who knew how to produce pain from these devices, and I wanted to learn rapidly. He explained that the machines, in the main, reproduced the effects of free weights. Free weights, Rob? Nothing to do with cost, it turned out – free weights are the simplest form of weights for gym training, being the short (one hand-use) dumbbell and longer (two hands-in-use) barbell – my learning journey was indeed well under way.

Rob explained that – especially for a beginner like me – the machines were generally a better choice as they are less likely to cause injury, especially once I understood the principles and safety features that applied both universally for all these machines, and specifically for the machine I was working on. Many of these principles also applied to free weights, I learned. And the correct term for training with either or both of free weights and such machines is resistance training, Rob explained.

The time passed in a whirl. Rob gave me an extra forty minutes on top of the hour we'd agreed, so I had almost my full hour with weights after all. However, the facts stopped being retained after a small portion of that. With so much information, much of what Rob went in one ear, out the other, and I needed to revisit them to hammer home the key facts. Jenny had one more day of work in LA before we flew home, and I decided my best use of that one day would be to learn more from Rob; not just learn more, but reinforce that first day.

We agreed that I would have a further hour of personal training time with him at Gold's the following day. He seemed pleased that what he had told me had sparked my enthusiasm and suggested, rather than just reviewing what we had just accomplished and showing me a few more exercises, that on that next day we could go further and create a resistance training programme for me that I would be able to follow once I had returned home. A programme consisting of weight values and repetitions; I could see spreadsheets and numbers appearing before my eyes – this was something that I saw working well for me.

The next morning brought a problem for Rob. A problem for him, an opportunity for me. Rob had planned to do some video work at Gold's after his personal training session with me, but his cameraman had let him down. Rob had the camera with him, and asked if I could do the filming instead. He said we would do a much longer session, and mix in his workout for the video with the time for my personal training. Probably take about three hours on it, he said.

I now realise that being able to watch Rob demonstrate and talk about each exercise, and seeing how the movements work together to train a particular body part effectively, was a remarkable opportunity; it was as if I was watching his future video on my laptop, except with the unique additions of the ability to ask questions once the camera was off, and for Rob to guide me as I then performed the same exercise that I had just seen through the camera lens. I was new to using a camera to record video, and I recall that much of my camerawork was ropey. We needed to do a few retakes. Rob knew I was an amateur in this aspect, just as I was in the resistance training itself. He was able to coach me in the video recording as much as in the exercise. My enthusiasm was at maximum – I was watching a professional at work here, and all the while learning more about the worlds of gym-weights and gym-video; things that would feature heavily in my life to follow. Those three hours passed in the blink of an eye.

At the same time as juggling his mental script for his pieces to camera, and checking the lighting, background and my camera angles and sound levels, Rob was creating a resistance programme for me and providing the education and inspiration that are the twin key roles of a personal trainer. Not for the only time in my life, I found myself in a role reversal situation – I was unintentionally acting as the eager youngster, learning from the professionalism of a near-infinitely more qualified teacher – who just happened to be under half my age. That age thing wasn't a concern for either of us, but it helped me realise that you are never too old to start something new, provided you really want to do so – a fact that I hope you'll remember when you reach Part Two.

We developed a good working relationship that session, and after gym we had lunch at The Firehouse, a popular post-gym restaurant near to Gold's. This was a lunch without beer, but the absence of my favourite brew didn't bother me – I was still on a high from the filming and the words Rob had been using in the gym.

Over lunch Rob set down a written strength-training programme for me to utilise back home, all exercises that I had worked on during both gym days, with a set of logical progressions for each exercise. We also spent a long time on nutrition – Rob wanted me to increase my calories, but add much more focus on quality of food. He noted there wasn't much protein in my typical diet, and he wanted me to add a specific focus on that – one of a number of principles that I added to my nutrition strategy from that lunchtime discussion. The combination of the advice on improving the quality of my nutrition, with the few hours we had spent in the gym together culminating in his programme for me, were designed to help me succeed at that most difficult of fitness goals – that question from earlier; the ability to put on muscle while losing bodyfat.

We also touched on his own story. He explained he had moved from his parental home near London to LA to pursue his career in fitness, a risky move that so far was paying off. He wasn't just a personal trainer; he had a string of fitness and bodybuilding competition titles to his credit, and a large and active following in the fitness world. He created videos that had had millions of views online, was featured in many magazines, and had his own TV show on cable channels. Little did I realise at the time how much of that was rubbing off, and would reproduce in me in the years ahead.

As we parted – me to the hotel and then with Jenny to the Airport, him to plan his next day's filming – he told me that he had seen enthusiasm for the fitness project in me that he had rarely seen in others, especially of my age group. He knew that I would have no end of questions on training and nutrition in future, and offered to act as an advisor by email on any question that came up in my continuing fitness project. An offer I was happy to accept, and indeed I made good use of in the months that followed.

I realise now that those two gym trips had been possibly the world's best introduction to resistance training. Several hours of gym work in the best gym in the world, under the guidance of a top professional and contest champion. The vast majority of people who train in the gym are not lucky enough to have that kind of introduction, continuing education and ongoing inspiration. I appreciate how lucky I was to have found Rob through that receptionist's referral. And not only that, I had made a friend – a friendship that remains strong to this day, despite the years and miles that separate us.

We never did return to the location of that third tricep, though.

9 – The Year of Fitness

I did a lot of thinking as I travelled back across the Atlantic with Jenny. Rob had definitely encouraged me to add resistance training to my morning cardio, and had devised a programme for me to follow. But something wasn't quite right in my head. As I review it now, I realise that the weights routine that Rob devised for me had many things going for it, but one that was lacking.

I couldn't see anything wrong with the programme, not that I was qualified to judge, of course. It covered all the key body parts, and with a choice of exercise types. Despite Rob's preference for resistance machines for a newcomer he was happy to prescribe mainly free weights for me as (a) he could see from our hours together that I was sensible and cautious in my approach and good at following his advice, so therefore reasonably unlikely to injure myself, but also because (b) neither Rob nor I knew what machines were available in my UK gyms. His programme for me was realistic in terms of time commitment, so nothing wrong there, and finally it had logical progression of weights and repetitions that would present incremental challenges as I went on. So far, so good.

What was missing? It didn't have an end-point, a target. Sound familiar? It was a programme for resistance training which would continue until... until what exactly? I was already doing one fitness project without a specific goal, the weight loss, and I didn't feel that I wanted to add another one with the same obscure outcome. Blame that project manager mentality in me again. I am obviously the one who diverges from the herd here because the vast majority of gym-goers are able to train very happily for many years without a specifically stated goal.

So, I created a second project. More of a replacement project, I guess, since success in it would make me fitter, stronger and healthier, all of which are positive steps in the original project's aim to kick that doctor's prediction out of play for good. I would have my SMART objectives all nicely sorted this time; this new project would be based on achieving goals in body shape and strength, measured through a series of variables tracked regularly. And I would set a fixed period of one year, which would take me up to age 53.

This would be a year where my fitness objectives would become top priority, my 'Year of Fitness'. I think spending time with Rob had made me feel like I could travel down the road to where he was, at least for some of the distance. I had seen a small sample of his life and it looked good. No longer did I just want to move from obese to average. I wanted to go beyond average to being unusually fit for someone of my age. There was no chance of my standing on stage like Rob and winning a fitness modelling championship of course (the very thought!) but I wanted to move to somewhere for which comments of 'Chris? Oh yes, he's fat' would be replaced by 'Chris? Oh yes, he's fit'.

I decided that I really had twin overall objectives for this: to increase strength by adding muscle and improve health by losing bodyfat; and the best way of doing this is by replacing some of my fat weight with muscle weight. Those words of Rob's that caused the 'Oh, sugar!' moment were still very much in mind. Jenny had of course noticed that the three stone I had lost had changed my appearance. The spare tyre around the middle was definitely inflated less, which she thought good, but more muscle would improve my look even further, she said. Jenny was keen to progress her performance in triathlon and other sports, and decided that she would also increase her fitness over the same time of one year. We would grow fitter together.

As you know I had already cut out much of the low-quality food and drink (that was key to me losing my first three stone) but I stepped that up a gear and Jenny's participation made this so much easier. I did not need to worry that I hadn't been out for a nice meal with her that week since she didn't want the excess unhelpful calories either. While trying not to be antisocial with our friends we did cut down on less-nutritious foods. Sadly, I can't remember anything specific about the changes I adopted for that year on the nutrition front apart from a single, very big one.

The one very big change I mentioned that I definitely do remember is that Jenny and I cut out alcohol for the whole year. My beloved traditional real ale was out of my life for 365 days. Jenny was more a wine drinker but she also saw the benefits to her fitness goal of cutting out alcohol from her life for that year. It would have been very tough if one of us was 'dry' and the other not so, but following this path together with all the support we gave each other made it workable. I'm not saying it's anywhere near a health food, but sales of Diet Coke in our neighbourhood went through the roof that year. To my taste buds, it was actually an improvement over original Coke, notably so when compared to the taste of low-calorie, zero-alcohol beer or wine.

I started recording calorie, protein and carbohydrate inputs - more detail than I had logged before. I was beyond the notebooks by now, but this was still before the era of MyFitnessPal and similar apps. I started logging this data on spreadsheets and reviewing progress regularly. Excel became an important part of my fitness life and remains so today.

We also set ourselves an additional target. Jenny wasn't interested in a prize for her own achievements (getting a PB in a triathlon was fine enough for her), but we agreed that if I set specific fitness objectives and achieved them in that Year of Fitness, our family budget could run to buying something significant as a reward for me. I'd always wanted a small convertible sports car, so a Mazda MX-5 was agreed to be my prize for success. This was definitely the carrot rather than the stick approach.

I took seven exercises that Rob had shown me in LA and put the others on the shelf for a while, so that I could concentrate on a specific subset for my new project. The exercises I chose were all ones that Rob had demonstrated and discussed with me; and the hours I had spent in Gold's made me feel comfortable I would be able to perform them safely and productively without supervision.

I'm going to talk in detail about those exercises now. Don't worry if the terms are all a little vague or indeed mean nothing to you at the moment. I'll explain much more in Part Two, when it's your turn, but if you do want a sneak preview then the numbers in brackets are my exercise reference numbers, and you can see a video[1] of the relevant exercise by following the reference from the link shown on the last page of the book.

The seven exercises I decided to take on were in two groups:

- I chose three free weight exercises with dumbbells. For each of these my target was to increase the weight I could move over the twelve months while successfully completing a set of ten repetitions safely. I selected presses while lying on a flat bench for chest (C23); and for shoulders I selected presses while seated upright (D11). For biceps, I selected concentration curls (A44).

- The other four were body-weight only exercises and for these the objective was simply to increase the number of repetitions I could do before giving up. These exercises were wide-grip pull-ups (B71) and close-grip chin-ups (B51), both primarily for developing back muscles, the close-grip ones also working the biceps. Third, I used dips as a triceps with chest combination exercise (A71) and finally I added sit-ups on a decline bench (M11) to work some of the abdominals.

After a few weeks, I decided to add more exercises as I noticed that I didn't have anything for the substantial muscles in the legs and could do with more for shoulders. I added some extra exercises for those but I won't explain those additional ones in any detail here, as I didn't add them to the seven that I was measuring for this one-year project. But I'll go into detail on the various exercises I perform later in the book - promise.

I was still doing my morning cardio five days a week pre-breakfast – still forty minutes on the cross-trainer, still bopping to the beat of my music, and still adjusting the levels to keep the heart rate in that 125-130 beats-per-minute target range. I wanted to leave a decent time gap before the weights; so the resistance training session was later in the day, sometimes on the way back home from work (at the gym next to the office) or later in the evening near home. On more than one occasion I found myself in the gym in office hours when I should really have been working, a policy that I employed more and more in years that followed. I'm getting ahead of myself here, but that approach rather explains why I was invited to resign into early retirement a few years later.

My resistance training was not every day. My target was three times a week on non-adjacent days. The reason for this is, which Rob had explained, is that it takes time for muscles to recover after having been worked, so the same muscle group shouldn't be trained on successive days. As I think back on that today, I now realise that this rule probably wouldn't have applied, as I was only doing one or two sets of ten per body part, definitely not to the point of fatigue. And in case you are wondering, this rule against consecutive days doesn't apply to cardio, as that isn't a muscular development process, but a fat burning and stamina building activity.

About this time, Cannons gyms were sold to and rebranded as Nuffield. I was regularly spending eight sessions a week there: five morning cardio sessions and three afternoon/evening resistance sessions in both locations combined – one near the office and one near home. Jenny had also joined our local Nuffield to help her in her fitness-increasing plans, so we often went together at evenings or weekends. This was good mutually-supportive fitness activity, as well as bringing the benefit of an increase in time spent with my wife than heading to the gym on my own.

With eight weekly visits I was, if nothing else, getting value for money from my multi-location gym membership over that year. But did I achieve anything else? You won't be surprised that I had turned to Excel to record my progress on the seven exercises, and so I knew that I would achieve my first objective of getting stronger by seeing the numbers increase on that spreadsheet.

I had a second objective, of looking better, appearing less of a 'fatty' and more of a 'fitty'; and if not outright muscular, then whatever is the opposite of that 'scrawny weakling' term from earlier. I have yet to discover any reliable objective measure of looks, but I wanted some way of determining that aspect beyond Jenny saying I was looking more attractive. And it was obvious, thinking back again to Rob's comments, that in addition to the seven resistance exercises, my variables needed to include body composition factors.

The human body is composed in the main of fat, bone, muscle and water. Obviously, there are other parts, organs, hair etc., but on the basis that there isn't much you can do about those and that their weight doesn't change much, then it was the first four I needed to think about. I reckoned that to go alongside my weight, I needed to calculate and record my fat percentage, the percentage of that bodyweight that is bodyfat. I didn't at that time know of the close link between water and muscle mass, or the value of resistance training and certain nutrients to bone density, so fat percentage was the only aspect I tracked.

There are many ways of calculating bodyfat percentage, but definitely the easiest is with bathroom scales that measure this by using tiny electrical currents passed through the body. The technology involved in these scales is called bioelectrical impedance. I purchased one from Tanita that operates on this principle and shows a fat percentage figure in addition to overall weight.

If my weight was going down and my fat percentage was unchanged, then I was losing weight equally from muscle/water and fat. That's what I think I had been doing for those 18 months until my trip to LA. And if the weight stayed the same and the fat percentage was reducing, then this was good, since that meant that I was losing fat and replacing it by the same weight of muscle and water. Finally, if my weight was going down and the fat percentage was falling too, then I was losing a higher percentage of bodyfat, and I may have been putting on a little muscle as well; and this was the ideal scenario. Rob had explained that putting on muscle is much harder than losing fat so I was under no illusion that this would be a 1:1 replacement.

I started a spreadsheet to track weight and bodyfat percentage which I recorded daily first thing in the morning. Using the maths in Excel and the numbers from the scales, I had data not just on bodyfat percentage but also bodyfat weight and muscle weight data, although I didn't set a specific target for these. I can't recall why as it's the sort of thing I would normally have done.

I decided to add waist measurement as a final value to track to replace a rather subjective sense that my trousers were getting looser'. It was the same thing being measured but with some numbers to go with it to satisfy the numbers-geek side of me. Three body measurements there to add to my seven exercises - good, I like ten.

So, I had a whole bunch of numbers to measure and a trusty spreadsheet to hand. What did I succeed in doing over that those twelve months?

	Starting	Target end	Actual end
Overall weight, st-lb	15-0	12-7	12-4
Bodyfat percentage	25	18	17
Waist inches	37	34	32
Dumbbell chest press –10 reps	16kg	28kg	30kg
Dumbbell shoulder press –10 reps	12kg	22kg	18kg
Bicep concentration curl –10 reps	10kg	18kg	16kg
Number of wide-grip pull-ups	0	3	3
Number of close-grip chin-ups	6	12	10
Number of chest/triceps dips	15	30	25
Number of decline bench sit-ups	25	50	50

You can see it was a massive year on the numbers for me and massively enjoyable too once I had become used to the enhanced level of diet control. I had no problem in keeping to the exercise requirements, as I loved my daily cardio and my three-times weekly weights sessions. I needed no encouragement on that front.

Looking back now to 2009, I find it hard to believe there wasn't the odd occasion in that year when my nutrition was off. I suspect it was of course for Christmas and other family big days. But I can't think of a specific instance when I went way, way off track. It's fair to say that I was 90% good in the months between the doctor's warnings and going to LA and it's also fair to say that I was 99% good in that Year of Fitness.

I did indeed look very different. I had lost most of my fat and put on some muscle. The word sometimes used is 'toned'. Actually, there is no such thing. Being toned really just means a bit more muscle and bit less fat covering it. I had lost the best part of three stone in the year and that's almost six stone since the doctor's glum warning. My trousers had come down from a value of 42 waist (40 if they had stretched a bit) when I received that doctor's warning to 32. I had an estimate of 40% as my bodyfat percentage way back, but, as the numbers show, it continued to come down in my year of fitness as my strength went up.

I was done. My year of fitness was a success. Jenny loved the new me. The numbers showed that I didn't quite achieve my targets on all ten variables, but it was enough to end that project and my fitness-focused lifestyle for good.

But of course, I didn't. As you'll read in the next chapter, I did ease off the accelerator pedal a bit - that's not the one in the MX-5, of course. However, devoting myself to my own fitness (and eventually helping others with theirs) was to become a permanent feature in my life.

And I know an Oxfam shop with a supply of size 34 and above trousers.

10 – The Ten Principles of the New Normal

The end of 2009 marked the conclusion of the Year of Fitness. I had completed it successfully and was now where I wanted to be. Time for a new project, perhaps? I remember evaluating the options I had for going ahead:

1. Roll forward the Year of Fitness, and try to continue in the same way, with the same intensity and focus that I put into the Year of Fitness. Who knows where that might lead? Move over Rob, perhaps?

2. Move into a maintenance mode, where I would aim to maintain my level of fitness but not strive to improve my fitness levels. Spend more time on the rest of my life.

3. Give up on the fitness idea, after all I had reached all my targets, and I was no longer on the doctor's watch list. There's food and beer a-plenty out there!

Well, which did I do?

Answer – none of them, well none exactly as written. Why not? None of them really appealed to me as a suitable plan for the way forward. I wanted a route ahead that I would embrace for the rest of my life or for at least as long as possible.

Thinking back, I had put a huge effort into the Year of Fitness. I didn't want to do that forever. I had forgone some fun non-fitness times during that year, such as a few parties missed, a number of drink-ups not attended, and I was keen to return to my favourite beers. I wasn't going to do that for good. So that's option 1 out.

Option 3 was a non-starter. This would only have been a valid option if I was following my fitness life to meet a specific objective as ordered to do so by the medics and if I was doing this fitness thing because I had to. But (remember the Magic Moment) I was doing it because I wanted to and indeed, I very much enjoyed it. Doing something you very much enjoy and is also good for you at the same time scores a treble top in my opinion. So, lets kick that option into touch (sorry, mixing my sporting metaphors here – and I'm a not a sportsman either).

That leaves option 2 – maintenance, that is to say moving myself from the overall objective of getting fitter to a new objective of maintaining fitness levels. This would mean not trying to make further progress into fitness and it would be about easing up and enjoy doing new things that my enhanced level of fitness would allow me to do. It would be time to throw away targets and thinking about goal-attainment, more taking time to make the target lines on the Excel graphs into horizontal lines.

Tempting - but perhaps not. Having had those targets for the Year of Fitness had spurred me on and made me realise that I actually am happiest when doing something constructive, progressing. I concluded that I didn't really want to stay where I was, even though I was far more fit and healthy than I had ever been. Sticking with my current levels of performance would have been a great example of maintenance and a relatively easy option for me.

I've heard it said and no doubt you have too, that 'if you're not progressing, then you are going backwards'. I thought about that a lot. Did it apply to me? It is certainly true for the youngsters because if your performance at 26 were the same as it was when you were 16, then you would be going backwards. Most people could improve on any fitness measure over those ten years. But it isn't true for those in their second half-century. If a fifty-year old can lift a certain weight in a gym exercise, run a specific distance in a given time or do a stated number of press-ups, and if that same fifty-year old can then deliver exactly the same results at age seventy, then I would definitely call that progress. I was in my early fifties, so I could easily convince myself that maintaining my numbers was progress based on that last approach. But, as I said, I wasn't happy keeping numbers the same. I didn't want option 2.

And I wanted aims that covered more aspects of my life rather than just the gym and food. I wanted some possibilities for activities that had no target numbers for a change. This was a redefinition of life within maintenance as applied to me. Nothing would have a target date, so it was my intention that this would be my approach to life that would continue until the grim reaper came for me or something else devastating happened. Get lost, SMART.

It wasn't to be a project. It would be a new approach to normality for me, principles that described a way of living that stretched beyond the kitchen and gym. It's an overused word, but it certainly applied to me: I was defining a new lifestyle that I would live from that point on. Going back to those three options at the start of this chapter, I suppose I ended up with a blend of numbers 1 and 2, plus a little bit of 3 as well.

What does that lifestyle look like? Welcome to the ten principles of what became the New Normal way of life for me, a term I use that defined key parts of my life back then, and continue to do so today.

1. Continue to make fitness an important part of my life, but **beware of going to obsession levels**. Try to progress on everything, but do so because I want to. It is way past being fit to meet a doctor's instruction. It should be fun activity, but keeping a sense of perspective and a feeling of balance. Do more of other activities that I enjoy and have no fitness relevance at all like spending good quality time with Jenny and friends. Fitness is indeed my main hobby but not my only one.

2. Carry on **eating and drinking sensibly** for most of the time. Don't go on a diet at any time but instead eat in accordance with these principles. I've set down an 'ideal day' of nutrition - details coming in Chapter 12 – and I keep this in mind during each day. I make it second nature so that it doesn't need conscious thought to know what is ideal and when I'm heading away from the desired track. But absolutely don't tell myself off if I vary from the ideal, even by a long way, provided that (a) it doesn't happen too often, and (b) I enjoyed myself doing it.

3. A typical day would have between **sixty and ninety minutes of exercise**, which would comprise some cardio, some resistance training and a little stretching. Any more than that and I'll be heading towards obsessed rather than enthusiast, and will face an increased risk of injury. I decided to log details of all my exercise sessions, so that I can see that my New Normal approach is allowing me to progress over time as the numbers improve.

4. While away from home on business trips or holidays I will do what feels best. I've already proved I'm good at finding **exercise opportunities away from home** and have long believed that if there's something you really want to do, you'll find a way to do it, and if there's something you really do not want to do, you'll find an excuse not to do it – another one of my favourite sayings. It's not an obligation for me to go and do a workout in a hotel room or beach. I probably will find a way of exercising because it would feel weird not doing so.

5. You knew there would be some numbers in here somewhere, here they are. At this point, my weight had settled down to 11 stone 7lb (161lb, 73kg) with a bodyfat percentage of 14%. That gives me a BMI of 23, and I like how those numbers makes me look and feel, so I have **committed to them to be my long-term figures**. I allow myself a band of up-or-down by two pounds on

the weight, and I need to increase the emphasis or 'turn up the dial' on my exercise and nutrition if I move outside of that four-pound weight band or above that 14% figure. I don't mind having a lower bodyfat percentage than that of course, but getting a lower number isn't something I specifically aim for. Lastly on the numbers, I wear size 30 or 32 waist trousers, and I'd like to remain there too.

6. I'm aware that fitness can be a bit of a solitary activity, so I actively look for things to do that are in accordance with these principles that include Jenny. She needs no encouragement in sports, and I will make sure that we **do more sport activities together**. I'll talk a lot more about that when we leave the gym in Chapter 21.

7. Thinking of what Rob has achieved, I should look to **do other things in fitness** such as writing articles, videos, travel, website, giving personal training, mentoring, radio, TV, attending expos, motivational speaking, devise courses, maybe even write a book one day. If it is interesting and I would enjoy it, then go for it; and take opportunities when they present themselves.

8. I picked up a massive amount of fitness ideas and tips from Rob. He told me how much he enjoys passing this information on to someone who will listen and benefit from it. I would like to pass on my own advice and experiences to anyone that is keen to learn and share in the joy of increased fitness at any age. There's real enjoyment in **passing knowledge on to an eager audience**. So, I will pass information on too, to anyone who is genuinely interested.

9. Never forget that my non-fitness friends may find all of this just a bit too much. Don't throw out all the 'Old Chris'. There are substantial bits of the Old Chris that were fun, nice and indeed loved by friends who haven't the slightest interest in fitness and

wouldn't know a dumbbell if they tripped over one. **Don't become a fitness bore**, in other words. I suspect I may well have been one in the Year of Fitness. That's just as I shouldn't be boring on trains, flying, beer and the other things I do.

10. I **shouldn't stress if I wander away from these principles for a time** because all of this is meant to be fun, and fun forever, not meant to be onerous. I don't need to make money at fitness to pay the mortgage, so I shouldn't treat it in the same way as work. A happy man is a very different person from an unhappy man. I'm definitely the first type. Life is finite – better to spend it cheerfully than miserably.

I need to own up to something. I am actually writing down those principles for the first time today, a little over ten years after I decided to use them to define the future normal lifestyle for me. So, these principles are actually being committed to written words today with 100% hindsight, and I hope without the benefit of rose-tinted spectacles. What I am writing today is what I believe today is what I would have wanted to write had I written it back then. I think that last, rather ugly sentence summarises it. It may make more sense on a second reading.

The ten principles state how I have been living over that decade and how I intend to continue. I have had ups and downs over this time, occasionally when my life has veered away – and you'll read about some of those times in the following chapters – but I always come back to this, the normal approach for me; and that is exactly what the normal is for anything of course, that state to return to when a situation has veered away from it for any reason.

Finally, I always take time to appreciate how far I have come – from the obese exercise-hater knocking on the door of some serious medical conditions back in 2006 to being fit and enjoying life though fitness today. I've kept my weight and bodyfat percentage at around the levels in these principles since then and my blood pressure, aerobic capacity, cholesterol and blood sugar levels have been back in the happy range whenever they have been tested during the past decade; and I have regained my flying licence. I feel much better about myself mentally - more confident and more positive for the future, and the belief that it's never too late to try something new is deeply rooted in my psyche.

What 'new somethings' did those ten years hold? For the remainder of Part One I will review what being fitter and less fat has enabled me to do. You will see how my life has changed since those early days of no exercise, poor nutrition and low self-esteem. I'm going to start by explaining the approaches to exercise and nutrition that I applied as part of applying my New Normal to me, and then I'll describe how I measured success from then until now.

11 – Training Approach

My view on training has changed remarkably little over the decade since my Year of Fitness. I've added some exercises and taken some away from time-to-time, often due to different equipment being available at the gyms I use. I've changed jobs a few times over the years and always moved my training to a gym near the new office, as well as keeping a gym near home as my regulars. And I've added more gyms for variety and for working out with friends or clients.

You may remember from my New Normal lifestyle that I like to exercise for between sixty and ninety minutes each day. That's Monday to Friday and I usually take the weekends off as pre-planned rest days in my workout and exercise plan. Sometimes if I've missed a key workout I can catch-up at weekends. Also, if I'm overweight and over fat compared to my targets, I may well do gym cardio at weekends as well, but both of those are the exception rather than the rule. I need my rest days!

That slot of 60-90 minutes is actual exercise time, not travel time or getting changed time. This is made up of three elements: morning cardio, afternoon/evening resistance training and an abs and stretching segment that can be anytime. Let me talk about each.

Morning cardio: My HIT and MISS workouts:

Early morning is the time for cardiovascular work where the focus is on using up energy and burning bodyfat. In the days when I had a proper job, I used to do my cardio at a gym close to work, before getting to the office. I described that back in Chapter 5, and the general principles didn't change: early train to London, perform my cardio exercise, then shower, suit and tie, pick up a nutritious breakfast and then in the office by 9am or not too long after. Now I no longer have that kind of job, so I'm free to go whenever I want; but I still go for cardio first thing.

Why so early? Since I don't eat beforehand, the body cannot use recently consumed calories for fuel during the gym session. It therefore has to turn to the other source, previously consumed calories that have been stored as bodyfat. I am extending my overnight fast until past the cardio. Such a prolongation of the overnight fast is the optimum time for burning bodyfat. I will have black coffee beforehand. The coffee has zero calories and the caffeine is a stimulant to help speed up the metabolism in order to burn extra calories; and as a side benefit caffeine encourages fat cells in the body to open up and the contents used for fuel. It's a win on many fronts.

There are at least two theories on fat burning and cardio. They both work and one may be better than the other on any individual. I do both to ensure I cover both strategies. These are what I call my HIT and MISS workouts. HIT is my slight abbreviation of HIIT – High-Intensity Interval Training. I shortened it by one 'I' to make it easier to pronounce, and so it goes nicely with MISS, which is training at Medium-Intensity Steady State.

Why two approaches? It's all based on heart rate and beats per minute. Intensity refers to heart rate, and the percentage of a person's theoretical maximum heart rate being used in the exercise. Opinions and calculation methods on maximum rate and intensity numbers vary, although the simplest calculation of that theoretical maximum number is 220 minus age. Do you remember the ideal range of 70%-80% that I mentioned earlier? Most sources agree that a heart rate of 90% or more of the theoretical maximum is exercise at a high intensity, while low intensity is at 60% or below. So, I call that mid-point of 75% my value for Medium Intensity.

Why don't I base my cardio on that high-intensity number throughout? In summary, at higher percentages the body tends to use a greater proportion of muscle mass as fuel and a lower proportion of bodyfat. I am trying to lose bodyfat here, not muscle. And at the other end of the scale too much at a low intensity means there's scope for harder work to be undertaken to achieve greater bodyfat utilisation. Not many fat-sourced calories are being used up for the time involved if the work is done steadily at a low intensity.

My MISS sessions are 40 minutes on a cross-trainer keeping my heart rate at a steady state through medium intensity exercise, that steady state being 75% of my theoretical maximum heart rate. Since it's impossible to keep to an exact number, I try to keep the rate within 5 bpm of that maximum. To save adjusting the resistance constantly I check only on the minute and make the change then if needed.

HIT is my approach on those early morning sessions on Monday to Friday when I don't do MISS, of course. HIT takes the cardio activity to the treadmill. It cycles the heart rate up and down from high heart rate to low and back again, and does this repeatedly for the full duration, which for me is 30 minutes. The theory behind HIT is that calories are burnt based on two factors: (1) the actual work being performed and (2) the heart rate. For the first, there's no real way to do more work without, erm, doing more work. So, the additional part of this theory concentrates on the second part, where I can benefit from excess calorie use without doing extra work, but from manipulation of the heart rate.

More detail: As I start performing extra work (such as going from walking slowly to running quickly) then the heart rate rises accordingly. It rises relatively quickly. Once I stop running the heart rate slows down to the resting rate, but it returns to that lower level much more slowly. This excess burn as it slows down post-exercise is the higher heart rate that leads to the extra calorie use. Ten seconds after switching from a fast run to a slow walk, I am not burning many calories from the current exercise, but my heart rate is still high, so the body is burning extra calories without doing the work to cause that higher rate. As a result, more calories are burnt than just the exercise would suggest.

To make this effective over time I repeat the process. A series of intervals is created. I run fast for two minutes, my heart rate rises quickly to match it; then I walk slowly, heart rate drops slowly to match it and keep on walking until heart rate is down to 65% of theoretical maximum, then I start again. By repeating these intervals, a number of these excess-calories-burnt-without-working-for-it sessions is achieved.

As I mentioned I eat nothing before my Monday to Friday morning 30-minute HIT or 40-minute MISS apart from getting a significant caffeine hit with a black coffee or two, plus water of course. And caffeine in the coffee helps increase the heart rate too. Many of the fat burner supplements work by doing just that, with caffeine often the primary ingredient. Once the cardio session is complete it's time for my power breakfast to break the fast.

There are more details of my daily cardio HIT and MISS in Appendix B if you want to see the exact speeds and settings I use.

Afternoon/Evening: My resistance workouts

The morning sessions are the cardio element. Here come the weights.

My resistance training workout can start anytime between 12 noon and 9pm, and these days the exact time depends on whatever else I have scheduled for that day. I choose to avoid the morning as I want a few hours recovery time from the morning cardio. I definitely wouldn't go straight from the cardio session straight into weights (or vice versa) as I wouldn't be able to give my full energy to both.

Back in the era of full-time employment I often did my resistance training in my lunch-hour. If that didn't work, then maybe on the way home from the office or later in the evening at the local gym after I had arrived home. My preference was for the lunch-hour as that didn't use any of my post-work time.

Each workout takes around forty minutes of in-gym time, including some warm up time and appropriate rests during the session. Thinking again of my office days, you can see that with a few minutes walking to and from the office, changing and showering, then the lunch-hour would indeed have to be a bit elastic. It often was, and I managed to get away with it regularly, until – well, until I didn't.

I gave my resistance training system a name – ABC7 – as it's based on the alphabet and, as I'll explain in a minute, there are seven exercises in each workout which is specific to a body part. The system has the following five workouts based on five areas of the body:

- Arms
- Back
- Chest
- Delts
- Elevators (Legs)

The first three are obvious and Delts is short for Deltoids, the anatomical name for shoulders. What about Elevators? That's the word I use here for legs because having reached D, I had to have an E in there to satisfy my sense of order.

As it's a bodypart-specific plan, the idea is to do only exercises that work the chest on a C day, the same for legs on an E day, and so on. In fact, it's impossible to isolate to that degree. You use legs if you are carrying dumbbells around to use on the Arms day, for example, and many back, shoulder and chest exercises involve arm muscles too. So, it's more to do with focusing on the body part mentioned rather than absolutely excluding everything else.

Days of the week aren't rigid, but I try to do five days per week, getting one each of ABCDE per week. In the perfect world, my ideal sequence is BCEAD across the days Monday to Friday. The reason is to use the big muscle groups first (Back, Chest) and then the smaller muscle groups at the tail end of the week (Arms, Shoulders). Legs are usually after two days giving the upper body a mid-week respite. It's a good principle to let muscles recover for at least 24 hours between resistance workouts (48 is better) and this body part split works well to preserve that idea.

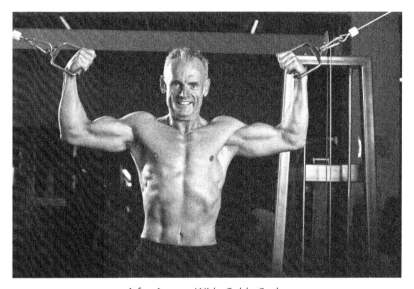

A for Arms – Wide Cable Curl

How about the weekend? Just as with the cardio, I take a break at weekends from this workout routine. But as I mentioned at the start of this chapter, if I have missed a day in the week for any reason, I could catch up on Saturday or Sunday and do the missed workout then; but that depends on what else Jenny and I are up to at the weekend. I would never do two of the ABC7 workouts on one day in an attempt to catch up. I would be tired from the first, and wouldn't have the physical energy (or the daily-renewed enthusiasm and freshness) for a second resistance workout that day.

Why seven exercises per workout? Muscles are in groups, and I want to ensure that I work each muscle within the group, and from all angles, to ensure that each targeted muscle is activated and does some serious work during the session. Creating seven exercises for each muscle group, in other words, for each workout, does that.

It also neatly fills the time available, originally designed to fit my work lunch hour, and I'm still with that timing now even without a clock-watching boss to be concerned about.

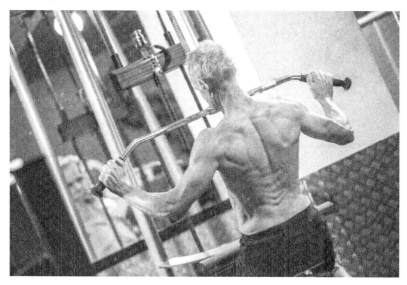

B for Back - Lat Pulldown

Some terminology now. A repetition (known as a 'rep') is a single movement that can, as you can tell from the name, be repeated. Pushing a weight up and then lowering it to the starting position is a single rep. And a 'set' is a group of repetitions performed one after the other with no break between reps but a break at the end of the group of reps before the next set, or next exercise. For most of the exercises in my workouts, I perform ten repetitions per set and three sets of each exercise. If that makes sense so far, then you'll agree that my target is 30 reps per exercise (3 x 10); and, taken a stage further, 210 reps per workout (30 x 7).

But I think here is the right place to explain why I record the data. I'm keen to improve my performance over time. I explained at the beginning of the last chapter how I like to improve over time, seeing progress in what I do. It's now over ten years since I first lifted a weight in a gym and I wouldn't be happy if I was performing any exercise with the same number of reps and the same resistance as when I first did it, even though I could justify a keep-it-the-same approach if I wanted to

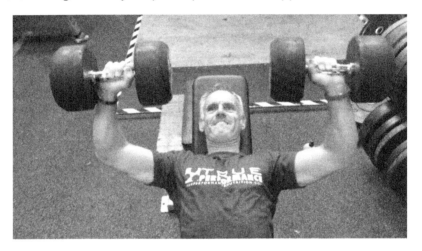

C for Chest - Incline Dumbbell Press

by saying that I'm ten years older. After all, it is indeed progress to still be able to do what I could do when younger. But no, I'm in competition in the weights room. I am in competition with myself, and my performance last time I did that workout is my only competitor.

Monitoring progress is therefore one reason why I record the data. There are two more; firstly, it's an incentive to continue. It's an easy activity to measure because there is a counting of reps and amounts of weight or resistance involved – all numbers. Remember that what gets written, gets done and what gets measured, can be improved – two more from my library of sayings. I have a single sheet of paper per workout showing all the exercises I did for that workout and my performance last time I did each exercise. That to me is the challenge of the workout.

The second reason is much more prosaic. You have already seen that I do 35 different exercises in a perfect week, seven exercises for each of five different workouts, ABCDE. However, I have multiple alternatives for most of my exercises, so I am not always doing exactly the same thing. There are at least three options for each exercise.

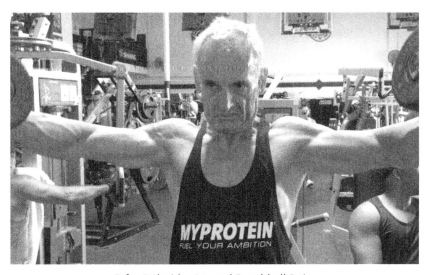

D for Deltoids - Lateral Dumbbell Raise

Appendix F lists all my exercises. They are prefixed by the letter that indicates which body part and therefore the workout and relevant day. All the Chest exercises begin with C.

The second character is the particular focus of an exercise. For example, the C1 group are all press-type exercises that target the upper chest. Within that group there are a few different choices denoted by the third character and I can select any from that list – it's C11 to C15. So, I will do one of those exercises (3 sets of 10 reps of course). And I will do any one from the C2 group, any one from the C3 group, and so on up to seven exercises for my C workout.

It's the same principle of other days – A, B, D and E. Legs exercises begin with L (not E), as I chose not to use my Elevators name at this level of detail. Finally, exercises beginning with M are for abs and are covered in the next section.

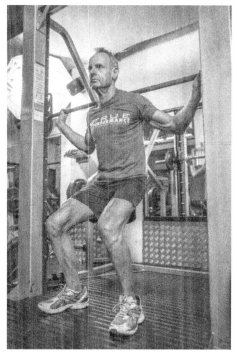

E for Elevators - Smith Machine Squat

Any two 10kg dumbbells will perform the same regardless of manufacturer, of course. That doesn't apply to the resistance machines, as each manufacturer has their own designs and different gyms favour different brands. Even exactly the same model of machine in two different gyms can perform in a dissimilar way, depending on how worn it is and how frequently and how recently it is lubricated or serviced. So, each gym/exercise/machine model combination needs separate tracking for me.

I've stuck to old-school when it comes to writing down my resistance training performance. I have a sheet for each of my five workouts, the exercises listed as the leftmost column and a column for each day to write in my performance by hand. Simple stuff and, you may be thinking, ripe for recording on an app on a phone or tablet. I tried that, but I prefer pen, paper and clip board. Why? It is one less thing to worry about. I've seen phones broken in the gym or left behind on the floor, or excess time taken to input the data. It's a lot quicker to fill in the relevant cell on my sheet of paper with a pen. Cell? I do use Excel to pre-format the sheets to be written on into a helpful grid. But that's it as far as Excel is concerned on recording the data because the actual numbers go down by hand.

One point that you may be thinking is – hang on, Chris has been doing these weights exercises for over a decade and each time he goes he tries to improve on performance. Surely, he can lift a house by now?

A good question, and indeed I can't lift a house, but I can, on most exercises, perform that same number of reps for about double the resistance compared to when I started. I think that number would be higher than 'double' had I started lifting weights when my body was able to adapt and grow much more quickly.

All of which would have been fine, if I had first visited a gym in my twenties rather than when I was over fifty, which, as you know, is when I did start. Progress was more rapid (less slow would be a more appropriate term) in the earlier years, but now I very rarely have to increase resistance to a new level on an exercise.

And there have been other reasons for non-continuous progress. For example, sometimes I've been injured or ill which of course knocks training for six for a short while, maybe just for one body part if I can still train other body parts that circumvent the issue.

Of course, performance improvement is not potentially infinite, particularly as the years pass. I know there are some heavy weights on the right end of the dumbbell rack in the gym that I'll never get close to, no matter how many more years I train.

But perhaps the predominant reason for non-continuous progress is that I sometimes choose to rebase an exercise by going back to an earlier weight. I do this when I feel that I am no longer performing an exercise 100% correctly. Maybe I have stopped using solely the muscle targeted and, well, started cheating just in order to move the weight. When this happens it's time to rebase. If I'm cheating, it means the weight is too heavy. Doing any exercise properly is more important than pushing the numbers up, because doing it improperly can massively increase the chance of injury. This is especially true with a heavy resistance, which takes us back to setback number one. Don't just count the reps, Chris, make the reps count.

I make the full workout available for purchase – the ABC7 System – and that includes many more details and spreadsheets to print for data recording. Note that it is a level of resistance training activity well beyond what I recommend for the Fat to Fit at Fifty plan. More details are on my Personal Training site.[2]

Anytime: Stretching and Abs

This third segment of daily training is for stretching and the core mid-section muscle group, the abdominals, known to everyone in the gym as abs.

This takes around 15 minutes, and I don't have a fixed time or location for it. The ideal time is straight after my main resistance workout of the day in the gym, but if I'm short of time (dashing back to work in the old days), then I can move it to another part of the day. It's not worth a third gym trip though. I've already been to the gym for cardio and resistance training, so if I don't do it straight after my resistance workout of the day (one of ABCDE) then I'll do it later on at home. This is the one daily workout that doesn't need equipment and I'm able to do it at home. It's only 15 minutes, ideally each day of the week, and I can do it while Huw Edwards is talking on the news if I haven't found time earlier.

The ideal is always straight after the resistance workout for a couple of reasons. The body is already warm and if there's a time gap then muscles become less flexible and the stretching will be sub-optimal in effect. Secondly, even though the session can be undertaken at home, the abs part has options to use equipment found in gyms. I'm a bit more restricted at home.

The 15 minutes divides into three groups of around 5 minutes each.

Firstly, I do a group of movement exercises called my 'Abs:100', a total of 100 reps divided into four sets, taking the first five minutes. You may recall that I said muscle groups need a day or two's rest between workouts. Well, that doesn't apply to abs. They are a relatively small muscle group at the core of the body. They have a good blood supply and are in regular use whenever you are walking or sitting, assuming you're doing that properly, and that means that they are fine with having a daily workout.

I can choose from a number of different exercises with M reference numbers (M for 'Mid-Section'). All are shown on my exercise list (Appendix F). The most visible part of the abs is the famous six-pack, visible on those individuals with an appropriately developed abdominal musculature combined with a low level of bodyfat. The first sixty of those reps are designed to work that area, a single set of thirty reps to focus on the upper part of the abs (any M1 group exercise), followed by a single set of thirty to work on the lower part (M2). On most people, the anatomical dividing line is about at the navel. The final forty are for the side abs, the oblique-line-shaped muscle on the sides of the middle torso. This means twenty reps on each side with half being leaning motion and half being a twisting motion. Both of those movements work that body part (two different exercises from the M3 group).

The second five-minute segment is to improve core stability and to help maintain correct posture. Unlike the exercises above, indeed unlike everything I've mentioned so far, these are static-hold exercises and no movement is involved. There are some options, but essentially all are variants of the plank exercise – holding the body still while tensing the mid-section (two minutes of an M4 group exercise, then one minute each side of an M5).

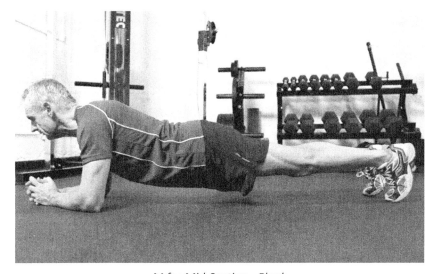

M for Mid-Section - Plank

The final segment is a range of static stretches. Designed to improve mobility, flexibility and balance, this is an area that too often gets neglected in workouts. I'm not neglecting it, I hope, by putting it in here – the final part of the final exercise period each day. Every stretch I perform is static rather than dynamic meaning that there is no bouncing to reach further. Go to the point where it stops being easy, then push that few percent further.

The stretches that I do are the ones I feel to be of most benefit to my particular situation at any particular time. If I'm recovering from an injury, then I'll modify the specific stretches that I perform in accordance with my rehab specialist's advice. For a few years I have used the services of a company called APS Coaching for this advice, and specifically their top rehab and flexibility coach Matt Lovett. His words are always wise and I have learned always to include Matt's suggestions in my stretching routine.

The stretches and planks are measured in terms of time and, as I mentioned, the initial abs session is performed as a fixed number of 100 reps. This suggests that I'm not in competition with myself for this third workout and that I'm doing the same every day, every week, every year. That indeed is true but I am consistently trying to improve my form on all three parts: to work my abs a little more thoroughly, to hold that plank that little bit steadier, and to stretch that little bit farther. But it is hard to measure, so there's nothing written down in terms of performance for this third daily workout. That differs from the first two workouts where I record the relevant numbers to encourage progress.

Summary

The approach to training described in this chapter and nutrition in the next work for me. I enjoy doing them and they are effective and are sustainable for me for the long term. I've been doing them ever since I adopted the New Normal more than ten years ago. I don't recommend them for everyone but, as you'll see in Part Two, a lot of the generic advice I give to newcomers to fitness over the age of fifty is based on what I did, what I still do, and what continues to work for me.

Let me go back a few chapters to the question that is probably the most frequently asked in fitness. Many people will say that it's impossible to succeed in both fat burning and muscle building at the same time. I disagree. It's not easy, but it is possible. To make it work I found I needed to have both the training and nutrition nailed and ensure the balance is correct between these two, not to expect instant results and to remain consistent in the approach; and make it sustainable in my lifestyle so that I choose to do it and do not do something else.

I've been using the approaches I'm describing here for more than ten years and in that time, I've kept my weight much the same but brought my bodyfat percentage down, which means I've lost bodyfat and added muscle. This isn't getting specifically into peak condition for a photoshoot or fitness model contest, something I'll talk about in Chapter 18, but this is more about raising my base line of condition that is that New Normal for me, the shape I'm aiming to be in all the time.

What goes with training to result in fitness-up, fatness-down progress? The biggest other component is nutrition, and that's next.

12 – Nutrition Approach

Having explained one half of my fitness life – the training – let's move to the other half, nutrition.

Like training, my approach to nutrition has not changed substantially over the years since my Year of Fitness was completed. The overall principles are summarised by the first couple of points of my New Normal approach covered in Chapter 10: eat sensibly most of the time, retain a sense of balance with the rest of my life, but attach a high priority to maintaining my fitness level. I'm sure you will want more info than that, so let me go into the detail behind that summary.

Let's return to when I met Rob for the first time, back in LA, when we had the first of our many long chats together. I was taking on board his advice on how I should change my approach to food and drink, as well as exercise, to accomplish the agreed twin objectives of losing bodyfat while adding muscle. For the first few years of being in the New Normal – I can't remember when the change took place, so it's going to have to just be first few – I was very enthusiastic following the advice Rob had given. He had developed a new daily eating pattern for me, comprising a full analysis of how many calories I should be having, at what times, and with what macronutrient breakdown. I followed his plan and used a spreadsheet (surprise, surprise) to record a check on progress each day.

Let's move forward to the second set of years. By this time, I was well established on where I wanted to be on weight and other body measurements. This was around 2014 and about the same time that I discovered the MyFitnessPal app for phones. Here was a tool that was a significant improvement on Excel for keeping a track of calories and macronutrients, since it was easier and more likely to be accurate than the spreadsheet. I used it from that day onwards, still do, and cannot imagine stopping. Bye-bye Excel – for this role, anyway.

A big innovation for me was to define two separate body states I could be in and understand that I would always be in one or the other. I describe those states as being within my Target Zone, or outside it. I've already covered these target values in point 5 of my New Normal principles, so as a quick reminder my Target Zone is defined as my weight being 11st 7lb (161lb, 73kg) plus or minus 2lb (1 kg) combined with a bodyfat percentage of 14% or below. I'll explain later about tracking these, but for now, take it that I measure these two values, overall weight and bodyfat percentage, first thing in the morning every morning and the results determine my state for that day.

Now I'll explain how my nutrition for the day changes depending which of those states I find myself in at the morning weigh-in.

Outside Target Zone

I'll start here with assuming I am outside the Target Zone on both measures; outside in this case meaning by being both over the Target Zone weight and over the Target Zone bodyfat percentage. This is by far the most frequently encountered outside-target state. After a few years of experimenting with what I eat and the resulting data, I have established the general principle that (a) the overall weight is changed by adjusting calories and (b) bodyfat percentage is affected by increasing the proportion of protein in my diet and amount of water. So usually, I would need to do both.

On these days I set myself a target of having consumed about 2000 calories by the end of the day. I know from experience that I will typically burn between 2400 and 2700 calories a day. That used to be an estimate but now I can confirm it as I use a Fitbit to track my activity.

That difference between calories consumed and expended per day usually leads to around one pound of weight loss per week in me.

Calories come from the macronutrients in food – protein, carbohydrates ('carbs' from now on) and fat – plus alcohol. MyFitnessPal shows the breakdown of the source of calories of each item that I eat or drink, so I easily have those numbers now. Life was so much harder in the spreadsheet days.

A general principle that I apply is to have more protein than most people, as protein is of primary importance in the building and maintenance of muscle mass. Along with that, I consume lower amounts of sugary carbs and saturated fats than most people, as calories from these are most likely to become bodyfat. The macronutrient ratio I aim for is 30% of calories from protein sources, 40% from carbs and 30% from fats. That works out to be 150g of protein, 200g of carbs and 67g of fat (don't worry about the maths there, it's in Appendix I if you want to understand it).

I track the protein and the fats. I don't worry about carbs because, very simply, if the calories, protein and fats are right, then the carbs have to be. Otherwise, it doesn't add up. There are two further items I track:

1. One type of carb that I track is sugar, due to its major influence on the storage of bodyfat. The limit I have is 67g. This isn't a round amount percentage of calories, but is achievable for me and helps control my overall sugars. It is also the same number of grams as fat, which is convenient.

2. One type of fat that I track is saturated fat, as many nutritionists believe that this is a particularly poor choice of fat due to links with cholesterol and heart health. I used to limit this to 10% of calories, but moved it down to 9% to bring it into line with published guidelines. It also gives a round amount of 20g.

That gives the five numbers I check: calories (2000kcal), protein (150g), sugars (67g), fats (67g) of which saturates (20g). Of course, these are daily maximum values, except protein which is a minimum value.

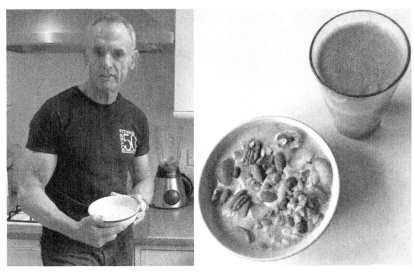

Preparing the Power Breakfast...   ...oats, nuts, berries, hot water and shake

I try to eat four times a day at four-hourly intervals, leaving a 12-hour overnight gap before I break my fast the next morning. A typical day would be a Power Breakfast at 8am then at 12 noon, 4pm and a final meal at 8pm.

If I can make the first meal an hour or two later, and the last one an hour or so earlier, then I will do so. Doing this will extend the overnight fast, the body's primary period for fat utilisation, from 12 to up to 13 or 14 hours, and it's good to be in a body-fat burning state for that extended time.

The third meal is in fact two half-meals; one half is a protein shake with some fast-absorbed (that is, sugar) carbs which I have straight after my main resistance workout of the day. The other half takes that meal up to a regular meal size for me. Those two halves could be timed together to make it a standard third meal, but the timing of the first half varies. It depends on the time of my workout, which can be any time after noon. So, I tend to regard my third meal as two halves: half after my workout, and half on schedule (4pm in that earlier example).

I don't carry daily surpluses or shortfalls over to the next day. I did this way back when I had a notebook and a target of 1600 calories – but now I treat each day as discrete. The reason for this is that 2000 is more generous, and also I am a bit stricter with myself to achieve it. That 2000 figure should be attainable without needing to borrow from the future.

The 2000 calories number is a firm goal as is the number of four meals (or rather, three plus two-halves). You see that an easy division is 500 calories per meal. However, the number of calories per meal doesn't have a hard number. If each of my four meals is between 250 and 750, and the total of all four is a maximum of 2000, I am happy.

The key to all this is planning. I have to know what my likely food and drink consumption is likely to be for the whole day, at the start of the day. I find it works best for me if I complete MyFitnessPal first thing in the morning, putting in projected eating for that day. At that time, I know when my client Personal Training sessions and other meetings are, when my workouts fit in to that plan, and if I have any social calories to accommodate. I can then build a plan that has a good chance of success for the day. Then all I have to do is follow it. This leads to another one of my favourite fitness expressions that I came up with a few years ago: 'Plan your eats, then eat your plan'.

What foods do I have to make this plan work? It does vary, and it would be tiresome if it didn't. I set out in Appendix C some foods that I try to have significant quantities of, some that I try to have average quantities of, and some others that I minimise. That list will also be referred to in Part Two of this book, when, yes, it's your turn.

As an example, here is a sample day's eating (and activity) for me on a day when I am outside my Target Zone:

<u>Typical day if Outside Target Zone</u>

Here is a sample day. To recap, my aim for such a day is to consume 2000 calories with at least 150g of protein and maximums of 67g of sugar, 67g of fats including 20g of saturates.

If you want to follow the numbers, for each meal I give five figures, first the total calorie amount, then a value for grams of protein, grams of sugar, grams of fats then grams of saturated fats. I'm actually outside my Target Zone as I write this, so it's convenient that I can use real data; what follows lists what I consumed on the day before I wrote this chapter.

Numbers are rounded and based on figures on nutrition labels and in MyFitnessPal. Often these don't add up accurately, but are close.

- The first thing, around 7am, is a black coffee. Zero calories, to provide caffeine as a stimulant and help promote bodyfat burning as fuel. Since there are no calories it doesn't count as a meal.

- Then it's off to the gym to start the HIT or MISS cardio, then shower and home. Keep well hydrated during and immediately after the cardio, probably around a litre of water in total, mainly afterwards.

- At around 9am, it's meal one, a Power Breakfast. This is based on oats with hot water with berries and nuts. See the photos and I describe it in detail in Appendix D. It includes a half a litre of whey protein shake with a single scoop of protein powder made with water. *(540/32/10/21/4)*

- 12 noon was time for meal two, lunch. As an example, it could be spaghetti carbonara with mixed vegetables on the side, followed by a low-calorie yoghurt, plus water. *(453/30/20/6/3)*

- I went for resistance training at 2pm, which could be weights. Drink another 0.5 litre of water. On leaving the gym, increase the protein with a two-scoop low-carb whey protein shake and an apple, which is the first half of meal three. The fruit could equally have been a pear, plum or small banana. *(252/38/11/4/2)*

- Part two of the afternoon, maybe at 4pm. This could be a high-protein, low-sugar snack bar if you happened to have a sweet tooth. You can almost convince yourself it is a normal chocolate bar. Many manufacturers and flavours are available, as an example here are the numbers for Grenade 'Carb Killa' Bar in Dark Chocolate Mint flavour. *(214/22/1/9/5)*

- The final meal is perhaps at 7pm. This was beef and ale stew, with some small amounts of bacon, plus more mixed veg, followed by a treat of a calorie-controlled chocolate mousse. *(537/69/25/12/5)*

- I always have lots of water throughout the day. There are two pints as part of my two protein shakes and two more accompanying my workouts, plus whatever further water I feel like. I have black tea and black coffee during the day, and maybe one (maximum) zero calories soda, all drinks with no calories, no macronutrients.

That adds up to 1996 calories, 192 grams of protein, 67 grams of sugar, 51 grams of fats of which 18 grams are saturates. These are numbers that are within my target of 2000/200/67/67/20. A lot of this calculation and measuring is estimation, not only by me but also by the manufacturers, so it is not as accurate as those total numbers suggest. There is a full breakdown of nutrition for that day in Appendix J if you want more detail.

What about the other conditions which lead to being out of my Target Zone? These situations occur much more rarely in my life, but, in summary: if I'm under target weight then I'll follow the Inside-Target protocols described next, but will increase the calories to a higher level than that given below; if my weight is within the Target Zone but my bodyfat percentage needs reducing then I can both increase the bodyfat-burning cardio I am doing every morning and cut down the percentage of sugary carbs and saturated fats, correspondingly increase the percentage of protein, and ensure I am drinking enough water. That usually does the trick for me, but as I've said, it's rare for me to need to make those adjustments so I won't go into detail.

Inside Target Zone

As a reminder, an inside Target Zone day is one where my weight, as measured first thing, is within two pounds of 11 stone 7 pounds (161lb, 73kg) and with a bodyfat percentage of 14% or under.

As you perhaps expect, these are less strict days than the outside-target ones described above. I still use MyFitnessPal, and record and check and record my calories there – and I am happy to go up to 2500 calories per day. Having tried that number for many years, that seems to work for me to keep me within the Target Zone.

Another change is that I don't calculate or record macronutrient numbers while inside the Target Zone. I do make a conscious effort to eat more protein than most people, and fewer fast (sugar) carbs and saturated fats than most, but I don't check these or record the numbers or percentage by macronutrient. As you know I do my macronutrient (source of calories) calculations if outside the zone, but that's a bit of admin I'm happy to forego as a small reward for being within the zone. The only daily input number I will log is the total number of calories.

I try to maintain the four-meals a day, at four-hour intervals, 12-hour overnight fast principles too. But I don't try too hard. I'm more flexible on that, especially if going out and spending social time with family and friends. This inside-zone time is when I can follow guideline 3 of my New Normal approach and occasionally let myself enjoy some quality time without thinking about the fitness implications. This is when the rules become guidelines or suggestions. I will decide if I want to follow them or not. I will, however, try to ensure that if I vary a long way from the rules, then it must be worth it. It's not worth blowing the day's 2500 calories or high-protein goals for some really rubbish food, cheap supermarket sliced bread or low-quality wine or beer. Make it good quality stuff, artisanal craft produced bread, for example, or an interesting ale from a craft brewer. In other words, make it worth the diversion.

I haven't logged a sample day when I'm inside the Target Zone, but many elements are much the same as the outside zone typical day above. Pre-cardio coffee, Power Breakfast, post-workout and afternoon snack would likely be the same. Lunch and dinner could be bigger – and of course there's room for some wine and beer within the extra 500 calories. What does that do the macronutrient split? Not a great deal of difference. I'm still high on protein, but I don't actually measure or track it, so when I'm in the Target Zone, calories are the only thing I count.

Conclusion

This is all beginning to sound a bit 'over-good', so let's be clear; I still have many meals out both for business and with Jenny and friends. I don't do fitness to have a miserable life. I do it to contribute to an enjoyable life. I let the idea of balance, as described in the first couple of points of the New Normal guidelines, apply on a regular basis, and these days I never turn down a social meal opportunity because of concerns over nutrition, even if I am outside of the Target Zone.

I enjoy working out how I can ensure that what I consume on these occasions is a nutritious option and I take account of what I eat in these situations in my nutrition calculations for that day. I rarely find I can't obtain something healthy and tasty in any type of establishment and still be sociable. An example was a couple of weeks ago I went to that old favourite, the fish and chip shop, with a group of friends, while actually outside my weight/bodyfat Target Zone. While some had haddock and chips, and others chose cod and chips, I selected the other combo – haddock and cod – and sliced open the batter on each fish to eat only the white meat inside.

I still enjoy the alcohol of course. The difference is that today I ensure it is all quality over quantity. You know that I am a passionate believer in beer and visiting quality pubs, but now the pints I drink are always special – no standard cooking lager for me. Of course, the volume has come down and I probably drink around six pints in an average week now, about the same as on a good day in the past … or do I mean a bad day?

You may have noticed that I use the words 'about' and 'around' a lot in my nutrition. That's because much of this is approximation even with MyFitnessPal to hand. Especially if eating out, where the ingredients and amounts have to be estimated. I've spent a lot of time reading labels over recent years and I've become good at estimating the relevant numbers for each meal.

At home, I am very lucky in that Jenny has now caught the nutrition bug too. Indeed, I think this whole transformation of my dietary approach would be impossible if I was concentrating on eating healthily and she wasn't. However, as a runner and triathlete, she is as keen on eating good quality and nutritious food as I am and, as a result, eating well at home isn't a problem.

I rarely feel the need to stray from my nutrition approach. I think my palate has changed to enjoy the more subtle flavours of, say, asparagus, veal and halibut rather than white bread, cakes and chocolate.

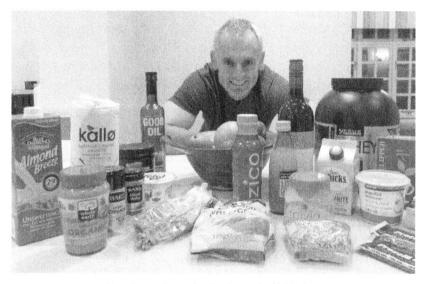

New ingredients in the household kitchen

Eating is totally different for me comparing today with ten years ago. I now know the effects on the body of various types of protein, carbs and fats, and the nutrition analysis table is now the first thing I look at on any new supermarket food item. Although my knowledge has improved, I still have much to learn. For example, I'm still unsure of the difference between a yam and a sweet potato, or what broiling is.

A key change compared to the past years is I now enjoy cooking and eating tasty and nutritious meals that I have prepared at home, as well as making the correct choices when eating out. As I am happy to admit, I am far from a cooking expert. But I do now know how to create something enjoyable and nutritious from some basic, quality ingredients to replace that staple of beans on toast, which was about as far as my culinary skills went in the old days. And talking of those old days, when I look back at Chapter 1 and read my old eating habits, it makes me feel like I am writing about someone else. Was that really me?

Everything I've mentioned above is what I, and most others, would call standard food and drink. I haven't mentioned anything that is anything that is a specific sports-related supplement. I exclude protein shakes from that category here for reasons you will discover soon. I'm no real expert on such supplementation and am willing to admit that. But if you want my views on this final component of what is consumed, then some brief thoughts form the next chapter.

13 – The Supplement Element

People often ask me about dietary supplements and which ones I take to help develop my physique to the level I have. While most of my story is, I hope, interesting, this bit really is not, as in the main I don't use supplements.

Hang on Chris, you might say, how about those twice-daily whey protein shakes you've been having since you first saw a gym? They were all over the last chapter! Answer: I don't classify protein shakes as a supplement, because they are basic nutrition to me. Protein shakes have calories and of course protein is its own macronutrient. One protein shake made with water has on average 160-200 calories and 40g-50g of protein, plus a small amount of fats and carbs. It is a foodstuff so is part of my daily diet and not a supplement to it.

So, what does constitute a supplement in the Zaremba vocabulary? Let me start by dividing supplements into a couple of categories.

Firstly, there are dietary supplements designed for the general public, by which I mean products that are not specifically targeted at the fitness sector, items you can buy at a high street pharmacy. If I am on a sustained period of calorie restriction, on my 2000 calories a day approach because I am outside my Target Zone, then I will probably have a standard multivitamin/multimineral tablet once a day just to make sure that I'm meeting the micronutrient needs of my body. In the peak of the winter or if I can feel a cold coming on, I'll take extra Vitamin C, a 1g tablet maybe twice a day.

The second category comprises the supplements aimed primarily at the gym-going community. There's a vast range of these, each brand and product with its own market approach and, I assume, significant marketing budget. You probably won't see these in most chemists, but probably some in specialist health food shops, certainly in dedicated fitness supplement shops and definitely all over fitness and bodybuilding magazines. I feel the manufacturers of these have identified that people who go to gyms are likely to be competitive to be the best they can be (like me) and will spend lots on anything which says it will help achieve that (which isn't like me).

The supplements range from pre-workout, in-workout and post-workout, and can be focussed on extra-fat loss, extra-muscle gain or extra-strength build, an increase in gym performance or any combination of those. As a group they have never really appealed to me because there is too much marketing and they are too far away from basic and natural nutrition and often very expensive; and are there really and truly no negatives to taking them?

There are a couple of exceptions to the part about my not using them. Firstly, a few years ago, Rob Riches started his own supplement company as he could see the fitness market booming. He saw the fact that dedicated fitness people are prepared to spend more than the average person, and he felt he could be successful at it by adding add his own personality and body image to his new brand. He asked me to test some, as he was interested to see whether the effects of his products on fifty-plus year olds were similar to those seen in his own age group.

That led to my first exception to the no-supplements approach. I decided to try one of his supplements, a fat-burner called 'Ripped', for two periods of about three months in the run-up to a couple of my fitness modelling contests, which you will read about in Chapter 18. As you might guess from the name, this is a supplement specifically of the fat-burner type; described as a metabolism booster and stamina enhancer, designed to keep the user going for longer both in the gym and throughout the day, burning more calories and using more bodyfat as fuel. Did it work? I'll let you know in a couple of paragraphs.

The second exception to my approach also occurred pre-contest, specifically in the period eight to ten weeks before those contests. These are the times when I was keen to progress to become the best I could be. My competitive spirit was turned to the max and, like everyone competing, I wanted to be in the best possible condition for judging and at show time. So, for, I think, four of my ten contests, yes, I took additional fitness supplements in the weeks leading up to the event.

I took two supplements in these periods: (1) Creatine, one of the best-researched supplements which is promoted to improve strength, build muscle mass and reduce post-exercise recovery time; and (2) BCAAs (Branched Chain Amino Acids) which are some of the building blocks of protein that the body needs and are said to aid muscle growth and reduce muscular fatigue. In summary, I took creatine and BCAAs supplements daily for periods of eight to ten weeks each before some of my contests, before two of which I also took the Ripped fat burner for the same period plus an extra previous month.

The big question is: did they work? Well, I lost weight, both actual weight and percentage of fat, and my gym performance was improved. Furthermore, on contest day I looked good with defined physique, noticeable muscle and low levels of bodyfat for each of those contests. But I can't guarantee it was the supplements that produced those results. As you will read in Chapter 18, I turned up the dials in both training and nutrition substantially before the contest anyway. Was it the Ripped? Was it the BCAAs? Was it the Creatine? Was it the extra training? I don't know.

When I look now at the photos of the other contests, those where I didn't use the supplements beforehand, then yes, again I have that defined physique, noticeable muscle and low levels of bodyfat. And If I compare the photos from all my contests today, I can't tell which were the ones that followed a supplement period and which were not. I would have loved to go back to Rob to tell him that I wouldn't have won without the Ripped, but I don't know whether that is true. I can't swear that it was the supplementation or the extra hard work on training and diet that made the difference.

Time for a general rumination. The fitness and bodybuilding magazines and online promotion in that market are full of adverts for supplements, in each case the supplement being promoted being shown alongside a fine photograph of a fitness or bodybuilding model, designed to make the reader conclude that it was the supplement being promoted that created that body that is seen. I've always thought that this is poppycock. The athlete depicted will be taking a whole cocktail of supplements (I hope including the one being promoted) and is probably spending way more hours in the gym than the reader being targeted. To suggest that the body shown is the result of taking that one supplement being promoted, a conclusion that is never actually stated but is the one that the advertisers want the reader to reach is ridiculous. However, I assume the adverts work as that type of marketing has been running ever since gyms and supplements have been around. No doubt the manufacturers will continue to prise money out of hopeful athletes based on their target market's optimism and belief in their imagery.

I can't talk about supplements without mentioning performance-enhancing drugs. One of these (I'll admit it here) is a product of which I am an absolute addict. There hasn't been a day in the past ten years that I haven't had my fix. I am at my local supplier practically every week for a new stash, often imported from Colombia or Costa Rica. It begins with C, of course.

As you probably realise, the C I'm thinking of here is caffeine, in the shape of coffee, and my local supplier is Tesco. Caffeine is a stimulant that helps alertness, fights fatigue, boosts metabolism and helps the fat cells release their contents to be used as fuel. Caffeine is a drug as it stimulates the central nervous system, and is indeed one that until 2004 was on the banned substances list for competitive sporting events if used in large concentrations.

The World Anti-Doping Authority determined that caffeine no longer met at least two of three criteria for inclusion on the prohibited list. The criteria for banning a drug are that (a) it has the potential to enhance sport performance (b) it represents a health risk to the athletes and (c) it violates the spirit of sport.

However, caffeine isn't completely in the clear. The stimulant remains on the Authority's watch list and athletes' caffeine levels are still actively monitored for patterns of use. Even if the ban were reinstated athletes would probably not have to abstain from coffee completely. The legal limit under previous restrictions was 12 microgram/ml in urine, which is roughly equivalent to drinking eight espressos over the course of a few hours. Nowadays caffeine is in such global use in every population that it is hard to believe it was a banned substance, but I think it just might become one if it was discovered today.

Finally, there is the world of illegal performance-enhancing drugs. It's a world I know little about and I don't particularly want to. I've chatted to people who take them, noticed people taking them (the changing rooms of most bodybuilder-focussed gyms is a key place) and seen the effects of them in people in the gym and on the stage. And I've heard stories of how such drugs have affected people in later life, assuming they are still alive to have a later life. At the very best, it's cheating; at the worst, it's suicide.

If you're looking for an exhaustive analysis of supplements on the health and fitness of someone of my age, then I'm afraid that this isn't it. As you've read, my personal experience of legal supplements is limited to just a handful of months of supplements that weren't really that extreme and my personal experience of illegal supplements is zero.

I believe that many people take supplements not to act as a supplement to an already very good diet and training regime but rather to partly replace the rigours of diet and exercise. 'I don't have to try so hard if I'm taking a fist full of supplements every day' is perhaps the mindset. This is not an approach that I endorse.

Instead, I believe that a supplement should be a supplement to a good regime. Ensure that the diet and the associated training are right and do that consistently for a significant period and you won't need them. That approach worked for me.

14 – The Scales of Truth

I have described the approach to nutrition and exercise which I have followed since 2009. Have I adhered to those always, every week since 2009? Of course not. There have been good times of holiday or visiting friends and bad times of injury or illness when they absolutely don't apply. But the key point is that I always go back to them following the interruption, whether that interruption was a happy one or sad one. The principles of my New Normal allow for that.

I try to stick to my approach whenever possible and practicable but I remember the other principles of my New Normal life too, those around life balance, doing what feels best and not letting fitness override other important aspects of life. I regularly review those principles subconsciously and without realising it, particularly the top four (review them yourself if you like, back in Chapter 10) and then I revert back to that normal state for me, using that fifth principle to guide me.

Again, going back to numbers, I keep to my plan on exercise and nutrition on about 75% of days. If I do veer away from the target numbers then I turn up the dial on both the food and training until those numbers are back where I want them to be, that is back in the that overall weight Target Zone of 11stone 7pounds (161lb, 73kg) plus or minus two pounds and with a maximum of 14% bodyfat. Although I like to exercise on holiday these are generally times when I give nutrition and exercise a lower priority than usual. Then it takes a bit of time to return to normal. Typically, it's a 2:1 ratio for me. If I've been on holiday for two weeks then I'll probably be outside the normal numbers on my first day back on the scales and it will take about one week to return to the Target Zone. I do work hard at these times.

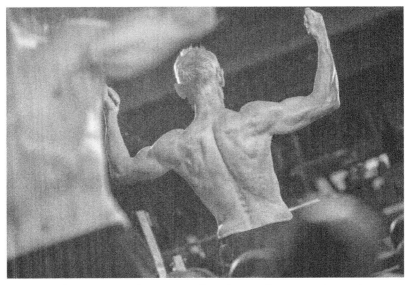

The mirrors at the gym confirm the good news on the scales

Consistency is such an important point. Even if I've eaten and drunk rather too much of the less-than-ideal stuff and undertaken far less than my normal amount of exercise and movement while away, I never feel as if I've 'fallen off the wagon', or that I've broken my self-imposed rules. I know I just need be a little more conformist than usual on exercise and nutrition when I return and I will be back where I want to be soon. These wanderings of the numbers outside of their Target Zone aren't a lack of consistency. They show how my plans for myself work to keep me where I want to be over the longer term. Consistency isn't a short-term thing.

Another not-short-term thing is keeping track of the data. As you would expect (you know me well by now), there's a spreadsheet involved. I've developed one which I have maintained on a daily basis since the start of my Year of Fitness, that is since October 2008. There is one row per day so I am now well into rows numbered over 4000 and I will reach row 5000 in June 2022. I have a minute on the scales in the bathroom unclothed first thing in the morning, every morning, and note down the numbers I see on a pad: weight, bodyfat percentage, water percentage, muscle amount and visceral fat level. Then I update the spreadsheet with those numbers when I'm dressed. I have a separate column for each variable. Of course, I don't take the scales with me on holidays so I have to fill in the gaps on the spreadsheet when I return as simple straight-line interpolated values between the last day before going away and the first day back.

There are a couple of calculations I've built into my spreadsheet so that I can see actual amounts as well as percentages. The percentages of fat, muscle and water should total close to 100. The remainder is bone, organs, skin etc. And similarly, the totals of weight of those three should be near to the overall weight. This gives a few additional calculated columns on the sheet.

I have of course (numbers geek that I am) derived a few different statistics and defined a few graphs from these covering several of the variables. Adding target lines to the graphs at the Target Zone weights and percentage bodyfat helps me to focus on and keep within those targets.

I mentioned a measurement for visceral fat earlier but didn't explain what that is. Visceral fat is the nastiest fat. It's not the fat below the skin that makes you appear fat but rather the fat that accumulates internally within and around the organs. You can't see it but it's the fat that specifically leads to diseases such as heart disease and type 2 diabetes; and clever scales such as the Tanita that I use can measure it. On the system that Tanita uses a visceral fat level of 12 or below is considered healthy, 13 or above is unhealthy. I am usually around 8 on this scale, plus or minus 1. I don't get concerned about this number unless it goes over 9.

I mentioned that I think the scales I use are clever and that is because of the significant amount of data presented in addition to just bodyweight. Figures are all given for variables including bodyfat percentage, muscle mass, bone weight and the visceral fat level that I just described. There's also a segmental analysis available on some models that has hand grips, and can calculate muscle mass and fat percentage on different parts of the body, but that is not a feature I use. I have enough data to manage with whole-body statistics.

There is one further feature that looks as though it should be very useful but I have found it has limitations. That is the calculation and display of metabolic age, a reading that shows how 'old' the body is based on body measurements rather than on your date of birth. The slight drawbacks in this are that some models seem to have a maximum difference of 15 years between the displayed metabolic age and real age, and others have a maximum value displayed for metabolic age of 50 years. If you accept and work within these limitations, then the numbers displayed seem reasonable.

One further point about scales and accuracy: I don't believe any scales are 100% accurate on anything, even if we exclude the metabolic age calculation. Weight is probably the easiest for them to be correct, other values have a lower level of dependability. For example, I've noticed bodyfat percentage can vary between two measurements only a few seconds apart. Another variable is that figures can easily change between two days depending on factors including how recently you've visited the loo. For this reason, early on in the design of my spreadsheet, I adopted a seven-day moving-average principle to even out the data and minimise the effect of any one-day spike in values in either direction. So, once I have entered today's weight (in pounds, such as 163) and bodyfat percentage in the appropriate columns for today's row, Excel will add those to the six values immediately above, then divide by seven and put the results in the columns that I use as that day's value and that the spreadsheet uses for graphs. I always regard any day's weight and bodyfat as these moving average figures, the average of today and the previous six days, computed automatically within the sheet. And doing this as a seven-day average means that any weekend variations are taken out as any day's figure includes every day of the week in its averaging approach. Excel is ideal for this.

A greater variation can be seen by switching to a different set of scales. I have found that even two instances of the same model of scales produce different results. For this reason, I only ever use the scales that I mentioned in the bathroom at home. I wouldn't take anything as a valid value from scales elsewhere such as in a gym. However, I do believe that the scales are accurate within themselves, by which I mean that if a lower figure is shown today than yesterday on any variable, then that value has indeed gone down. Perhaps the absolute numbers displayed may not be accurate but the direction of travel will be.

If the numbers that I record and that Excel computes for me are to be of most worth, then I need to eliminate all the factors that can pollute the data. One such is swapping to different scales that I just mentioned; another is changing the time of day that measurements are taken. Therefore, I use the scales once a day only and at the same time every day. Just after brushing my teeth and having a shave, to be precise.

I am not going to give you 4000 rows of data to look through (do I hear a sigh of relief?) but to show the overall effectiveness of my approach to life over the last decade I have just added a further calculation into my Excel sheet. It shows that I have been within my targets on my key weight and bodyfat percentage measurements on 75% of the days over the last decade. That's good enough for me and I believe it shows I have the balance about right.

In my mind the 'Scales' in the title of this chapter originally referred to the scales of balance and juggling my exercise and nutrition with the rest of my life to produce an outcome with which I am comfortable. But the word also refers to the much more mundane object on my bathroom floor. As you can see, I pay a lot of attention to both definitions.

15 – Pretiring into Fitness

You should have a good idea by now of how I spend a substantial part of my life. You've seen the training pattern I have adopted, and how my nutrition plan is structured and works alongside that training to help me achieve my goals. You've seen the way that I track and record my performance to check whether the nutrition and training are working together as they should so that I can meet my target numbers.

If you take all the time spent on those activities, in the gym, travelling, showering, shopping, cooking, eating, that is going to come to probably five or six hours a day. Let's put in eight hours on top for sleep, that still only covers fourteen hours a day. How do I spend the other ten?

Chapters 11 and 12 started by saying that my approach to nutrition and training hasn't changed much. Strategies on both are much the same today as they were a decade ago at the end of my Year of Fitness. That absolutely is not the case for the rest of my life and plenty has changed in those ten years.

What remains unchanged are the good parts such as being married to my wonderful Jenny and enjoying time with great friends with some decent traditional ale and enthusiasm over trains to share. What has changed is, well, pretty much everything else.

The first of those changes was in my employment. Until 2011 I was in full-time work based in Central London in the same business sector that I had been in for around thirty years, developing and supplying software to financial institutions. It was, by most people's standards, a good job. I had worked for six different companies over the years and was quite senior in a sales role. I regularly travelled the world to see prospects and clients sometimes business class and even, on a couple of occasions, managed to convince my boss that I needed to go on Concorde.

However, by 2011 the sector was struggling and so was I. The impact of the global financial crisis in 2008 hit all of the companies in the industry with very few clients wanting to invest in new software. Morale was low at all levels in the company that I worked for; and everyone was taking long lunches and a 'can't-be-bothered' feeling hung heavy in the air. I spent loads of time in the gym when I should have been at my desk and others made the pub their refuge. It was no surprise when the company wanted to downsize and looked to me to take voluntary redundancy. After some hefty discussions I managed to upgrade it to early retirement. That was the best business deal I had negotiated for years. I left the office early that year for the last time with a big smile on my face. I was not yet 55 - time to start the rest of my life.

I had no firm plans at that stage. I knew I wanted to spend more time on fitness activities because the gym bug was well entrenched by that stage. It took a few months of thinking before doing anything major; thinking about not having a boss, not having the daily commute, being able to do whatever I wanted. I knew I didn't want to be a layabout. Here was the opportunity not to regress but to progress further with my fitness, in some way. But which way?

Surely even a gym-junkie like me can't spend more than two trips a day to the gym, around 90 minutes a day. I know that some people do spend multiple times that but, no, I was happy with my workout plan (you've just read it: cardio first thing, resistance on a bodypart-split routine afternoons/evenings, stretching and abs later). That would stay as it was.

Jenny thought I should do something useful with my time. Not work as such, no boss (please, no boss), but not proper retirement. That can wait. I agreed with her. I wanted something before that, a halfway house between employment and being retired. How about pretirement? Thanks, Jenny, for inventing that word.

Around this time, Rob Riches visited the UK for a few weeks in order to see his parents and present a series of fitness seminars. Two of those seminars were at the gym-and-classroom facility that a company called Premier Training used in North London, and Rob was kind enough to invite me to attend. I knew much of the content already because I had been speaking to him on and off for a few years by that stage, but I learnt more, as I always do with Rob.

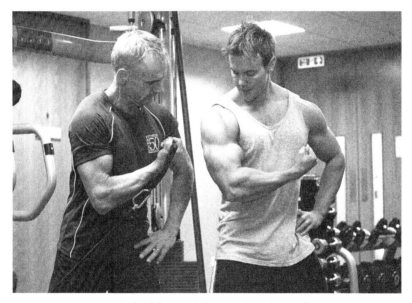

At a Rob Riches training seminar in London

One evening he paid Jenny and me a visit at home and I sought his advice on something more specific to me than was covered in his public seminars – how someone in their mid-fifties and with time on their hands should or could take fitness from the point I then was. We talked until late. Rob thought it was going to be just a social visit and I think he was grateful to be heading back to his folks at about midnight, rather than me rather forcing him to discuss my approach to fitness and life as we had for the previous few hours.

I remember something specific that Rob said late that evening, I think I can recall the words exactly even though it was seven or eight years ago:

> *'Chris, if you carry on in the way you are describing, then five things will happen – four good and one not-so-good.*
>
> *Firstly, you will continue to get fitter, but that is obvious. You will become exceptionally fit for someone of your age, especially someone taking exercise up later in life than most.*
>
> *Secondly, you will have a great time doing it. I know how this stuff makes you happy and it is going to continue to do so.*
>
> *Thirdly, you will meet some really nice people, especially if you look at fitness beyond you own exercise and nutrition and maybe see if you can help others in their fitness goals.*
>
> *Fourthly, assuming that you want to and that you make and take the right opportunities, you may become just a little bit famous.*
>
> *Finally, however, you won't make much money from fitness. It isn't easy making a living in this business. Don't ever think of it as a substantial means of income'.*

I was fully supportive and in agreement with all of Rob's ideas, perhaps not the fifth one, but I accepted that went with the first four and if I had really wanted to make significant income then the software industry is probably where I should have remained.

He could see I was lapping this stuff up, and offered to introduce me to John Shepherd, a man who combined being an athletics coach with being a magazine editor. Rob regularly wrote articles for John's magazine, UltraFit, and I suggested to John that I could write some too. John thought that an excellent idea. I was happy to do it for zero fee (perhaps that's one reason why he thought it was excellent!) and soon after that I was offering fitness knowledge and advice every month in print in UltraFit. John thought my regular column needed a title, something to tie the articles together, and the term 'Fitness Over Fifty' was born.

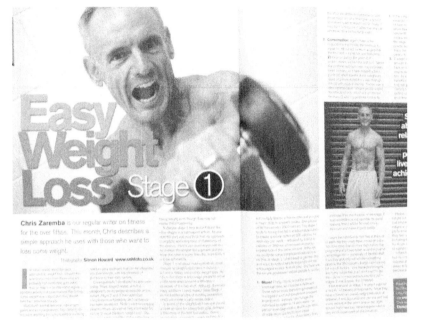

One of my articles in UltraFit Magazine

I penned the Fitness Over Fifty column in UltraFit magazine every month for over three years. I was content to earn nothing from it and was pleased with the publicity it gave me and with the satisfaction I gained from helping others both generally through the columns and specifically in the questions that were submitted from readers. Sadly, UltraFit as a magazine is no longer with us. Like so many magazines, it has been replaced in our habits by online activity; but I still occasionally bump into people who recognise me (or my name) from my monthly columns, and John and I are friends to this day.

I enjoyed writing those Fitness Over Fifty articles but, not long after the first couple had been published, I felt I needed something else to occupy my post-software years. Rob had mentioned the idea of a website. I knew nothing about building one, but I had time on my side and a bit of knowledge of IT, so I created my own site[3]. I was lucky that the domain name FitnessOverFifty.co.uk was available (the .com variant had been taken by someone in the USA), so I licensed that domain, arranged hosting and started creating.

I wanted the site to be a repository of information useful to someone who was now the way I was back then, so I stored information relating to fitness for the over fifties, both on nutrition and exercise. At the time I wasn't providing any services, so it wasn't a sales window, but it was a way of getting my views, recommendations and experiences out to an audience bigger than the readership of UltraFit magazine.

It took a few months before I was happy to go public on what I had created and now, several years after the site initially went live, it still takes time to maintain as I continually want to develop it onwards. I'll never be a whizz on HTML but I enjoy doing what I can; and it seems to be making an impression. Last time I searched on Google, typing in Fitness Over Fifty brings my site up first and the number of page views of the site is into seven figures.

With magazine articles and web site both well under way, what else could I or should I be doing to fill all this non-employed time? Well, I have always enjoyed showing others how to do things. In all of my jobs in financial software I was happy to take on the role of training new users in the systems developed by my various employers, or giving demonstrations of the functionality within the software we provided. And way before that you may remember from Chapter 1 that back in my sports-avoiding days at University I presented on the campus radio station. While there I was soon appointed to be the head instructor to help teach new recruits to learn how the presentation studio operated, a role I very much enjoyed. Now where is this leading? Combine instructing with the gym, perhaps?

I decided that I would become a Personal Trainer. I love being in the gym and I love helping people learn new stuff, and being a personal trainer would involve both. And I would earn some cash for it (not much, I remembered Rob's last point too); and although I don't want to give too much of an altruistic flavour to this, it would be something I could do for other people. If I could help people of my age group to become fitter and healthier and maybe avoid them receiving warnings like mine from their own GP's, then I perhaps I would be contributing a little to improving society too. I felt sure I could advise others who now are the way I was once, and could help them to derive many of same benefits from fitness that I've had; and I'd hope that they would have as much fun as I have had on the way.

Hang on. I knew a few personal trainers - Rob for one. And all the PT's I knew were much younger than me, and way fitter. Even with my new self, I was nowhere on the fitness scale to be compared with the average PT. Was there a market for a personal trainer of my age, by now nearer sixty than fifty? Would anyone employ such an individual? Did I want to be employed by someone, and hadn't I recently changed my life away from one with a boss, a move that had made me really happy?

Questions, questions. I didn't know the answers, but I was keen to find out. Jenny was right – retirement was indeed becoming pretirement.

16 – It's Starting to get Personal

Let's recap. I'm going back to 2012, aged 55, when I had recently taken early retirement from my job in financial software. It was still a novelty to wake up in the morning and not to have the one-hour commute into London. My fitness levels were very much were I wanted them to be because I was in the Target Zone on weight and bodyfat, and I was juggling fitness activities with the rest of my life to achieve a balance with which both Jenny and I were happy.

I had definitely been caught in the fitness lifestyle, keen to try new things that would expand my interest and, as you know, my thoughts had turned to becoming a Personal Trainer (PT). Jenny was fully supportive. She wanted me to find ways of occupying myself that were constructive and she helped me realise that I was still just a little young to hang around the house without a focus for some of the day (that would have been most of the day, apart from gym trips). I had actually reached that conclusion a long time earlier, but had not realised it.

Thus motivated, I planned my future as a PT, armed with enthusiasm and a cheque book. I soon discovered I needed both.

I had already decided that I would be an official trainer, one that is properly qualified and insured to offer Personal Trainer services. I had met a couple of unofficial ones, without formal qualifications, but they had seemed to be just guys that simply loved going to the gym and wanted an income from it. One even remarked to me that it was far better to operate in that way. There was no need to spend hours in the classroom and thousands of pounds on training courses, he said. 'I know how to lift weights!' was his final comment.

I rejected that approach quickly. I had decided that if there was a market for a PT of my age, and I was still decidedly unsure if there was, then the clientele I would be looking for would value official qualifications and an industry-wide standard of approval. A bit of research revealed that insurance is a big thing here. If a client became injured during a training session that they were paying for they could resort to litigation against the trainer. And if that trainer were unqualified, he or she wouldn't be able to have insurance to cover it.

I didn't realise it at the time but another factor is that most gyms don't allow a PT to operate on their premises, whether employed by the gym or freelance, without appropriate qualifications. And a further factor, which really only emerged as I put my business plan together upon the conclusion of my course, was that I decided to offer a top-quality service, which I would offer at high-end prices. The kind of clients I would want to recruit wouldn't even consider an amateur approach. They are used to buying quality, professional services where the skills and qualifications of the provider are impeccable. But how to judge the quality of a training course?

I learned that there is an industry-wide body ensuring standards in PT courses called REPS – The Register of Exercise Professionals. As an aside, I congratulate whoever devised that acronym.

The two most relevant standards here are the Level 2 award, a fitness instructor, the qualification needed to 'floor-walk' at most gyms, show people how to use the equipment and offer basic levels of advice on different exercises; and the follow-on Level 3, the standard award level for Personal Trainer.

I wanted a qualification at that level of accreditation so I decided to consider only courses being offered that had been assessed by REPS and awarded the Level 3 certification, somewhere that took the activity of teaching those courses as their key business with facilities and staff to match. I didn't need to look far.

I have already mentioned that on a couple of occasions I had visited the Premier Training facility in Highbury, North London, where Rob had hosted fitness seminars during his occasional visits to London. So even though I'd never attended a course there previously, I already had some insight into the way they operated.

The Premier Fitness approach ticked all my boxes, as the saying goes. They were well known in the training-of-trainers industry and their courses were well respected and of course REPS accredited. The gym in their Highbury location was dedicated to the practical side of the training of new personal trainers and went alongside several classrooms for theory sessions. They ran multiple courses concurrently with a team of full-time instructors. Every bit of their operation spoke of professionalism in what they did.

The only thing that concerned me was the commute. It was a 90-minute journey each way and although I had undergone similar daily commuting for most of my adult life, I didn't feel like doing it again. However, they explained that they had a local centre in Windsor, thirty minutes from my home, which didn't have a dedicated gym but did offer the same courses taught to the same standard and had access to the public gym in the same building. I was sold.

Their Level 2 course was of two-weeks duration and Level 3 a further four weeks. Both courses were on-site three days a week with home study online on Tuesday and Thursday. The first course is a prerequisite to join the second and I signed up for the full six-week block. I learnt that there were a number of additional modules that could be added later if I wanted to specialise further, but that six weeks would be enough to start me as a fully qualified PT and able to ply my trade wherever I could. I decided that the later courses could wait.

As you can see, I was keen, but I still had some concerns of which most were linked to my age. I hadn't been in a classroom for 35 years and I wasn't convinced my old grey matter would absorb facts as well as it had back then. And although I was fit for my age, I didn't know for certain whether my gym skills would be up to the level of the youngsters who would be learning alongside me. I thought that most of my fellow students would be straight out of school or college and have the natural strength and flexibility that goes with people of that age, especially those that are into sports and exercise. Finally, I was a little concerned about whether I would mix well with my classmates, as I expected to be old enough to be the grandparent of some of them.

I needn't have worried. The material was new to everybody. My age actually probably helped as I had more knowledge at the outset than some of the younger ones. Some of the subjects like anatomy, for example, were new to me, but others, such as nutrition, were subjects on which I had a fair knowledge through the years of making myself fit and listening to experts, including those seminars with Rob. The Premier course's combination of lectures, discussions and web-based home study worked well for me.

On the practical side, again my worries were groundless. Every student had more physical flexibility than I had and most would have more strength, but I had sufficient in both departments to show that I could train others competently. And I learnt that, to be a good PT, instructional ability, interpersonal skills and empathy are of more value than being able to reach your toes or lift the heaviest weights.

A final word on my classmates: on both courses there were a couple of others over forty but the majority were in their twenties or late teens. I was buddied with three much younger students – Chris, Sam and Katherine – and I found that the age gap added to a mutually supportive approach, each bringing different fitness experiences to share.

One plus point for me was that I was keen to learn, which surprisingly wasn't the case of everybody in the class. There was a small number of students who still behaved like the naughtiest of naughty schoolboys and had to be told off by the lecturers frequently. Hard to believe that this wasn't compulsory education here, they had each paid thousands of pounds (or their parents had) for them to attend. They didn't complete the courses and I suspect they are probably are offering unofficial PT somewhere today.

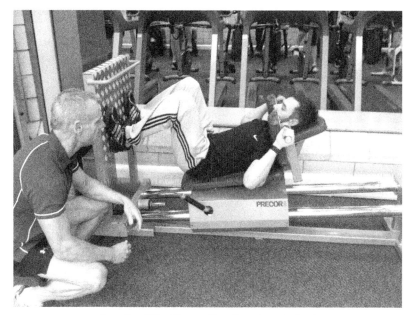

Practice PT with another Premier student

I did complete the courses and the old brain indeed worked well enough for me to pass all the exams. I added some additional courses from Premier in Advanced Nutrition for Weight Management, Advanced Nutrition for Physical Performance and Suspended Movement Instructor (which is being able to teach using the straps supported from above, such as TRX). With those additional courses I was awarded an upgraded qualification of the International Diploma in Advanced Personal Training, which is proudly framed at home.

That wasn't the end of my education as a Personal Trainer. There is something in PT, as in other professions, called CPD – Continuing Professional Development. It's the ongoing process that professionals use to refresh and renew their skillset. It is good both for reminders and also to extend knowledge in new areas, or perhaps for learning some techniques that just hadn't been invented when the original qualification was awarded. Points are awarded for additional qualifications earned, and already qualified PT's are required to maintain a certain number of CPD points over time.

I obtained my CPD points in the classroom and gym at the Premier location in Highbury and also online. Recently Premier moved to being an online-centred business and all of my recent CPD is undertaken online with them and several other providers. Whatever the location and whoever the supplier, the professional development of my PT skills continues.

I think I proved that I wasn't too old to start learning; I hope I will never be so old that I have to stop.

17 – The Personal Business

One of the learning modules of the Level 3 course is on finding employment and marketing yourself as a PT. I tried to remember the theory of those aspects of the course as I set foot in the real world and tried to determine how to obtain clients for my fledgling business.

A key point is that I didn't want to work full-time at this, or anything like it; a couple of hours a day would suit me fine. I was not counting on the income to keep the home going (and I remembered Rob's point five) and I saw this as a 'hobby-business' that would keep me occupied in my post-employed life and help others on the way. I was unusual in that aspect in terms of the Premier course, since most of the attendees on the Level 3 course were looking for PT to be their main income; but I actually don't know how many did. I know that Katherine and Chris moved to other things and used PT income as a side line but Sam stayed 100% with PT and now has a thriving business with his own Personal Training studio.

Qualified PTs fall into one of two camps, attached to a gym or freelance. Those attached to a gym may be employed or just contracted to be able to use it. Either way, there is a cost involved to the PT. If the gym books the clients for the PT the gym will take most of the cash; or if the PT takes his or her own clients to the gym, then the gym will require a rent payment of several hundred pounds a month, or the equivalent in terms of additional hours being a gym instructor (the gym floor-walker I mentioned before) or performing other employee-type tasks.

If you can detect that this doesn't sound like what I was after, you would be right. A freelance PT sounded better.

A freelancer can operate at home or buy a van and take equipment to a client's house. Also, with permission from the local authority he or she can give training in parks and the like. A further option is to negotiate with a gym for the freelancer to operate on a pay-as-you-go agreement, whereby every time the PT takes a client to the gym, an amount is paid to the gym by the trainer; and of course, the trainer builds that amount into the charge he or she makes to the client. Most gym chains don't like this arrangement, since it could be seen as depriving their own contracted PTs from getting business. But smaller, individually owned gyms usually consider it. In addition, there are PT-only gyms now opening for which the pay-as-you-go PT model is their only way of operation.

This pay-as-you-go approach worked for me and from 2012 up to today I offered it in a total of seven locations, all near home or in Central London. The benefits to me are many: I don't have to buy my own equipment, I don't have to get cold and wet in the park and I'm not committed to any overhead costs, because if I don't have a single client in a week, then I pay nothing. The drawbacks include having to do all my own marketing and source clients and the gyms where I have had this arrangement expressly forbid me from recruiting their existing members. That's fair enough, since that's a protected market for the gym's own PT resources, as I've mentioned before. Of course, the gyms need to view evidence of Level 3 qualification and relevant insurance. I would be very suspicious if they didn't want to see those.

One other way for a qualified PT to earn income is as a group instructor, taking classes in everything from spinning to yoga. Group sessions often work well in the park, too. I've thought about doing that and indeed, if the offering is right, there's more money to be made if ten people are paying you for an hour of your time rather than one. However, I've always preferred the one-to-one dynamic of individual training, getting to know the clients really well, building the rapport and the client's confidence in the trainer to know how to motivate them to help them attain their goals. My PT offering includes tracking a client's progress over time as well as some 'before' and 'after' photos if they want that, and I love being able to share in their happiness of a goal having been attained.

One early decision I made was that I wanted to work specifically with those aged over fifty. There were several reasons for this: Firstly, I could show them the changes I had made to my own life since being obese at fifty, and if I could do it, perhaps they could too. Secondly, I didn't think that there were very many PT's in my age group (most PT's were much younger) and competition between them for clients was perhaps greater. Next, I already had the Fitness Over Fifty name and website. And lastly, if I had clients in their twenties or thereabouts, they would probably be fitter than me before we started the first session together. While not being a definite reason for not proceeding, this would certainly be a less than ideal situation.

I thought more about the demographics. As I mentioned in the Introduction, over 50% of the UK adult population is now over fifty, and the majority of those are retired or entering a pre-retirement phase. These people are living longer, and seeking to maintain an independence from support and increased quality of life for those extra years. These are people who usually have more time available than before for leisure activities, and cash reserves are often high, factors combining to drive a keenness for fitness and life-enhancing activities. But I have found that often they are concerned over how to go about it, wanting to maximise the benefits and minimise any potential downsides. This applies to those who take up running or cycling to some degree, but especially so to those who turn to resistance training. That's when a personal trainer can advise, instruct and design a training and nutrition programme that takes into account any concerns or constraints the client has, and helps motivate them to achieve their goals.

I've found there are some differences in the way people either side of about fifty like to be trained. By 'like to be trained' I mean they turn to me for advice, which they follow while I'm with them during the training session of course, but also willingly follow when I'm not around. I've heard many times from the over-fifty clients that they did a session or two with another, younger, trainer previously, but didn't continue. I always try to determine why that is, so that I can ensure my own approach to them is one that will be adhered to for the long run.

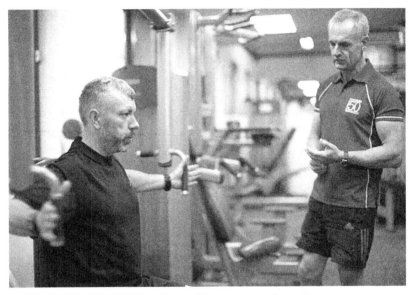

Personal Training with Sean - one of my clients

There are more likely to be medical issues or concerns to be taken into account with this fifty-plus age group. As their trainer, I have to remember and make it clear to the client that I have no medical qualifications and completion of the pre-activity medical suitability form and the discussion about it is a very important step. And that's both in detail at the start of our relationship and before each subsequent session. I'm more than happy to communicate with their GP if required, to obtain medical clearance, and am very keen to modify the exercises that we undertake to suit any constraints.

Progress tends to be slower with the over fifties. They also tend to require just a little more coaxing to try a new form of exercise. Older trainees also appreciate and accept the approach of continual but gradual progress over time, whereas the youngsters may want more rapid results.

I have found that older people tend to be better at following instructions both in the gym with the PT and outside by adhering to additional exercise and nutrition guidelines given as 'homework'. That homework is vital. A PT sees a client typically for one hour a week, which is way under 1% of the 168 hours in a week. The success of any client's fitness project doesn't depend on what the client does in that one hour. It depends on what they do in the other 167. It's the job of a good PT not just to think about the hour that they are with the client. They have to provide the tools and encouragement such that the client will follow the PT's advice until their next session together.

One particular aspect I've noticed is that older clients don't need to see new exercises or approaches continually. They aren't so likely to be bored by doing the same set of exercises for every session. There's a level of familiarity they like, and are sometimes a bit reticent of change. A typical Personal Training session could contain perhaps ten exercises and I would keep those ten in the routine throughout, changing one on average every four visits. Younger clients don't appreciate this level of repeating the same routine and need to be 'entertained' by regularly encountering new exercises. That isn't to say that the exercise routines I favour for my age group are the same each time. It is the same exercises but I increase the challenge by either adding more reps, slower speed or an increase in resistance. I'm a massive fan of Incremental Progressive Overload, the principle that progress on muscular development (and other aspects of fitness) is best made in very small increments repeated on a regular basis. This is even more true of the older client.

To show this to my clients, I keep a detailed spreadsheet for each client and review it with them before and after every session; and from this they can see their progress. I also calculate on the spreadsheet a performance factor as a percentage of the previous session. Typically, I like to be able to tell a client that their performance this time is in the range of 101% to 103% of their performance last time because this really adds enthusiasm. Going further, after a few weeks of training I can also compare the most recent performance as a percentage of their initial values. My clients understand compound interest principles and this does indeed keep their interest and enthusiasm levels up. Both this overall calculation and watching the numbers increment on each exercise over time isn't possible with a constantly changing set of exercises.

I find that the over-fifties client is happy to be numbers-driven in this way and is enthusiastic about reviewing the performance spreadsheet weekly. That same spreadsheet also shows body statistics such as bodyfat percentage and amount, percentage of water and metabolic age; and taken together this spreadsheet review is a key component of my personal training approach. One aspect where it helps is if there is a progress dip on one week for any reason; so, if the body statistics or exercise performance have performed less well than hoped for on one week, then I can show the continual trend from previous weeks and that usually overrides the initial disappointment.

This numbers-based approach, with the analysis that I do and share with my clients, is one that I think works much better with my age group than those younger. As you know I've been numbers-based on so many aspects of my own fitness, and perhaps it is my enthusiasm for that which helps my clients subscribe to that approach. I don't think those much younger would be quite as keen on reviewing spreadsheets and following my performance analysis from the accumulated data. That's a big generalisation, I know, and maybe apps are changing that.

I receive so many requests for personal training from this age group these days that I can't help them all. I've set up a network of personal trainers located around the country, people that I know personally and am convinced by their abilities to work with folk of fifty and over; and I try to pass enquiries I receive to those other trainers whenever I can. But it's getting busier all the time.

As an option, I also now offer Personal Training 100% online, which removes all location issues. My most remote UK client was in Wick, and globally it's Auckland! Using a video call I can develop a training strategy and nutrition approach that works with the client's domestic constraints and makes sure the client accepts the plans, accepting that they are reasonable and attainable. They have to 'own' the route to the desired outcome. A key thing about online is that it has to be long-term (at least three months) and the client has to commit to weekly online check-ins with me during that time. And that can be much more frequently than weekly if the situation demands it.

Back to face-to-face, and since 2018 I have been offering[4] Personal Training in three gyms: one in High Wycombe near our home, one in Central London (near Oxford Circus) and one in Islington, not far from where I started my Personal Trainer journey. I arrange my week to concentrate all London and Islington clients on the same couple of days to minimise the travel involved, and I usually catch up with an old friend or two between clients at lunchtime. That arrangement wouldn't suit everyone, but it works well for me.

My oldest client was Mike, aged 76. I had been training him for over three years and in that time his strength, flexibility, waistline, muscular development and cardio-vascular capability had all improved, as had his heart recovery rate and aerobic capacity. According to the metabolic age calculation on the body analysis scale I used on him each week, his body ended up ten years younger than it was when we met. He's happy to continue without my help these days, and I know he'll continue to progress.

Another client is Nick, aged 58. He's been kind enough to write about being on the receiving end of my Personal Training offering. That is in Appendix A.

 As you can tell, I'm a big fan of personal training for those in my age group, both in-person and online. I use the phrase that an individually designed training programme devised for a person aged fifty or above will add years to your life, and life to those years. I think I've proved that on myself, as the approach I use with most of my clients is the same as I use on myself, and that is perhaps the final point of why I turned fitness into a pretirement business. Getting fit worked for me. It helped me to move from being obese at fifty to becoming a fitness model champion at 55, and it continues to change my approach to health, fitness and just about every other aspect of life in my early sixties. I like to think I'm a good example of what can be accomplished and I'm sure my clients wouldn't choose a hairdresser who has a lousy haircut.

I could go on but I think I've been ageist enough for one chapter, so I'll leave it there. What was that bit about a fitness model champion, again?

18 – Taking it to the Next Stage

I continued to have holidays in LA, about once a year on average. I realise how lucky I was to be able to do this. Thanks to my pretirement, I had no regular job, and I was able to schedule my Personal Training client commitments such that I didn't see them, or saw them only online, during the week or two that I was away each time. So, I had plenty of time for holidays to schedule those trips to the USA.

Jenny wasn't so lucky as she still had a full-time job and had the constraints of annual holiday entitlement to juggle. She was happy for me to have some of those holidays on my own or with one or more of my fitness friends as she knew how much I enjoyed being in the Southern California fitness-focused lifestyle for those weeks. Of course, we went together on some of the trips too and those weeks with Jenny had a different emphasis with rather more eating out and being traditional tourists and rather less time in Gold's gym. I caught up with Rob on most of these LA trips, and on one of these Rob suggested to me that I should enter a fitness modelling competition. 'Like bodybuilding, but nicer' was a summary of his description of the event.

My initial reaction was that this was absolutely not for me. I told him that firstly I was way over fifty and I'm sure that everyone in these events would be half that age. Secondly, I knew I was unusually fit for someone of my age but I didn't think I had a competition-standard physique or anything like it; nor would I want to do whatever was necessary to make it so. Thirdly, I didn't have much of a competitive gene in me and I had spent most of my life avoiding competitive sport. I summarised those views by telling him that that wasn't for me. He smiled and said 'You will...' as we parted.

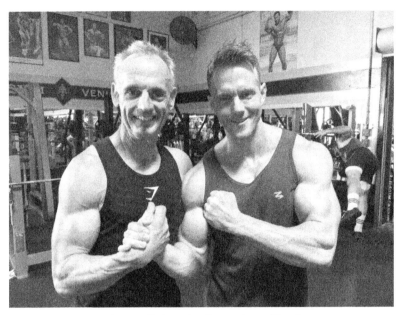

'You will...' said Rob over in California

Rob and I met again later during that LA trip and we talked on the same subject. I knew Rob was keen on physique contests for himself. He had what seemed to be a room full of trophies from such events and was regularly entering new ones; and it appeared he wasn't going to let me off that easily.

He pointed out that stepping on to the competition stage was a logical step in my new life, a step which would help in taking me from a Personal Trainer into more of a Fitness Professional. As we chatted, he gradually convinced me (or maybe I was convincing myself) that (a) I shouldn't doubt my abilities or condition and I really had a stage-worthy physique (b) there are contests with age categories so I would only be competing with my own age group (c) I would actually enjoy it, both the preparation and event itself (d) it would give a specific target to my fitness activities (e) it would look great on my fitness CV, and finally (f) he suggested I might actually win something if I just became a little competitive and tried.

So, there were six reasons in favour compared to my three against and indeed Rob had demolished my three within his six. I lost that argument but began to realise that I was happy to do so. Yes, he had convinced me. I decided to take this idea forward once back in the UK.

At home again I discussed it with Jenny. She thought this would be an interesting and exciting opportunity for me to try, just the once that I wanted to do it of course. I ran through the points in favour, which she agreed with and she particularly liked the one about being goal-focussed. We talked about this and noted that much of what I had undertaken on the exercise front had been towards a stated objectively-measured goal, reaching a certain number of somethings on a scale of something. The objective measurement is getting a trophy, ideally first. My fitness targets in the past rarely had a date and this time it would be different, a project which absolutely had a definite and non-negotiable end-date, stage day. I explained that I would have to be stricter on both my nutrition and training during the countdown to the contest and Jenny was happy for all that, so long as I didn't want her to follow the same, sterner regimes. I agreed.

I researched and discovered an organisation called 'Miami Pro', which ran physique events in – where do you think? – Miami, of course. No, it's actually a British organisation and the venue for their events is St. Albans; I guess Miami just looks better in the name. They were organising a show, their UK Championships no less, in April 2012 and as well as bodybuilding there would be categories for muscle model and fitness model.

I looked into both. There are similarities to bodybuilding in these two categories, but the muscle model category, taking this first, is a more relaxed look than bodybuilding, promoting muscle tone, body symmetry and pleasing appearance far more than outright size. And the fitness model category is one stage further away from bodybuilding. It's ideal is a fit and healthy look that is properly marketable within the fitness modelling and media world. I wasn't sure I fitted the definition of a successful competitor in either muscle model or fitness model categories but I was certainly closer to both of those than to a bodybuilder.

As well as categories for males and females as well as various ages, heights and weights, Miami Pro announced they were launching new 'Masters' categories for those aged fifty and over in both muscle model and fitness model. This would mean that entrants in these divisions wouldn't be compared to those in their twenties or anything like. I also couldn't decide whether to enter muscle model or fitness model so I decided to go for both, calculating that if I am to undergo several weeks of pre-show preparation, I may as well do this for ten minutes on stage rather than five. Before the day was out, my registration was in.

I told a few friends about my competing once I had registered for the contest. Some thought it was a joke at first (the fact that contest date was April 1st didn't help) but most were very supportive. I recruited one particular friend, Neil, to enter the contest in the same two categories as me. Neil and I trained at the same gym, and I guess we were probably comparable on stage, although he was a youngster at a mere 50 compared to my 55.

I decided to focus on the contest as a key priority for the period of eight weeks running up to the event – February and March. I decided to change everything that needed to be changed in my daily routine for those eight weeks to give me the best chance of performing well. Eight weeks may not seem a long time, but I was already good on my approach to training and nutrition; so this was a period of tightening everything up, improving each aspect by 10% to 20%, rather than a wholesale re-write.

Specifically, I decided this would be a no-baddies time on my nutrition. Anything high in sugar or saturated fats was out and I was back on the rule of no-beer (or anything else with alcohol) that I had last employed three years earlier in that Year of Fitness. On the food front I stayed heavy on the protein and fibrous carbs, and a typical meal was grilled chicken with some green veg such as broccoli plus maybe a hint of white carbs - a small part of a baked potato or small handful of rice.

In the gym I redoubled my efforts mainly by ensuring that I didn't miss a single day. My morning cardio was seven days out of seven, the afternoon resistance workout, the same. I made the leg workout twice a week, to give the upper body a rest for those two days. And to ensure I missed nothing I found a great local Personal Trainer, Russell Lee of Reel Health and Fitness, and saw him at his gym at Pinewood Film Studios twice each week in that run-up period to the contest. Yes, I knew how to lift weights, and yes, I was indeed a PT myself, but adding a further pair of experienced eyes to the mix helped me ensure I missed nothing and would be able to concentrate on any weaknesses in my physique and presentation. Russell's guidance was invaluable.

I mentioned presentation and that is the final element. It is good to have a contest-ready physique but less good if it can't be shown to advantage when it counts. I repeatedly practised my walk on to the stage, getting into the poses, smiling at the judges, then finally standing at the back of the stage, still on view after my turn and potentially influencing the judges' opinions even after my turn at centre stage was over. So many competitors in these events, I learned, spend ages getting the training and nutrition right and don't even think about presentation before the day of the event. I wasn't falling into that trap. If the mirrors in our house or Russell's gym had run on batteries, they would have required regular replacement for those pre-contest weeks.

Rob advised me that one thing I should do close to that day on stage would be to have some professional photos taken while in that peak condition. He introduced me to a UK-based friend of his, professional fitness photographer Simon Howard. Rob happened to be in the UK at the time so a date was chosen close to contest day and I duly met Simon and Rob in a gym in Colchester for my first ever fitness photoshoot. I'm not quite sure why we went to Colchester as the location wasn't particularly convenient for any of the three of us, so I assume it was selected because it was a dedicated gym facility that we could have just for ourselves for that afternoon.

I'd had a couple of sessions on a sunbed in advance of the photoshoot. I looked more post-August beach-holiday than the near-snowman colouring that I would otherwise have had on that March day. It was indeed fine for the photoshoot. However, I learnt that my new colouring was nothing compared to the dark shade I would need under the harsh bright lights of the stage.

Rob and Simon coached me in the best positions to be for photos to be taken. Often the positions he chose for a shot included using weights or other items of gym kit. Simon and Rob had both been through this photoshoot process many times and they knew how to position lights, reflectors, gym equipment, camera and me to optimum locations for each image. All this was totally new to me and yet again in the fitness game I was learning something totally fresh and fascinating from people half my age.

Simon sent me the final images a few days later. They were very well composed and his posing instructions had indeed succeeded in making me look like a true fitness model professional. Simon is a true master of his art. All of the non-stage, quality photos of me in this book are by him.

As I mentioned, a skin tone of a much deeper shade of brown was needed for the contest itself than for the photoshoot. The tan makes the muscles stand out more, the separation between them being more evident, shadowing is more obvious and the skin tone has to compete with strong stage lighting. All the pre-contest information I had picked up suggested that the darker the tan, the better. If it looks ridiculously dark at home it will be about right under the stage lights.

Luckily, the sunbed shop near where we live offered spray tans. I scheduled a visit the day before the contest. I knew spray-tan day would come and I wasn't looking forward to it. Definitely one of the weirdest feelings, being sprayed all over (not quite all over, small trunks were worn) such that thirty minutes after starting, by the end of the second coat and on conclusion of the hot air drier cycle, I was a deep mahogany colour. The sprayer enquired before the final application if I was really sure I wanted it that dark. The enquiry told me that I was on the right track to meet the suggested colour requirements.

I felt very self-conscious walking home from the tanning salon. In accordance with their recommendations, I was wearing loose fitting clothing that I didn't mind getting colour on and I had prepared our bed at home with old sheets and duvet. I hoped for two things during that walk: one, I didn't meet anyone I knew and two, that it wouldn't rain. I turned out I was lucky on both counts.

Off to St. Albans the next morning. Stage time came four times for me on the big day; twice for Fitness Model and twice again for Muscle Model; once for each category to do a theme-wear with costumes (I chose private pilot) and once with a series of poses front-and-centre of the stage together with comparisons where I would share the stage.

I knew it would be a scary, wonderful, unforgettable once-in-a-lifetime experience. I had no idea how the judges would regard me but of course, I wanted to do well, both for myself and for those who had helped me reach this point – my fitness coach through all this Rob Riches, my recent PT Russell Lee, and most of all Jenny – all of whom had pushed me to attain new heights I didn't think I could reach.

I'd been through the nutrition, the training, the walking and posing practice, and the tan. My numbers on show day were good – 11 stone 6 pounds (160lb, 72.5kg) and 9% bodyfat. In summary, I think I handled everything correctly in my preparation.

That crowd of friends I mentioned earlier came along with Jenny and Russell to St. Albans to wave banners and cheer me on from the audience. I had every incentive to perform well.

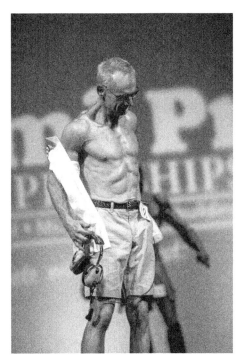

Somehow the pilot shirt came off

Each time my turn on stage came around I looked into the audience to where I knew Jenny and our friends were seated, but I couldn't see them. The lights were too bright and the auditorium too dark. But I could just about see those judges in the first few rows, and gave them everything I could: tense the biceps a bit more, squeeze the abs a bit tighter, flash the smile a bit wider. All of the tips I had from Rob and Russell were forgotten, but by that stage my plane was on a joyous version of autopilot and just doing what had become second nature as a result of my weeks of practice. I couldn't see them, but could hear my support group calling for me and cheering me on.

It was a unique and exhilarating experience and not once did I think how daft this situation really is: standing on stage in a theatre with not very many clothes on at all, spray-tanned to levels way beyond reasonable, being viewed and evaluated by hundreds of people and with multiple cameras recording every move. Nor did I ponder the ridiculous ratio of months of devotion and effort that went into this compared to the few minutes of on-stage time trying to impress the opinions of the judges.

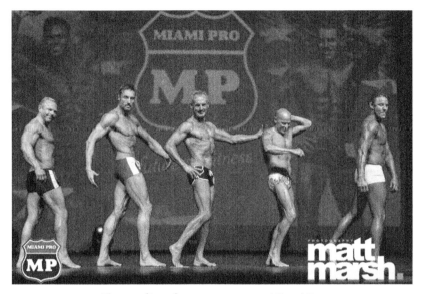

The top five of my age group at Miami Pro

At the conclusion of the evening of the Miami Pro UK Championships, I was a happy and grateful man: happy to be awarded runner-up in the Over Fifties Male Muscle Model and winner in the Over Fifties Male Fitness Model; and grateful for all the love and support from Jenny and all the help and encouragement from everyone else that had made this once-in-a-lifetime experience so successful for me.

Two Miami Pro UK Championships trophies came home with us that night, one runner up and one winner, and an envelope. The envelope contained an invitation to compete in the Miami Pro World Championships six months later. Today the UK, tomorrow the World?

You know what I said about once in a lifetime... well, that wasn't to be the case. I bet you're not surprised.

I competed in that World Championships later that year, and then a further three Miami Pro events in the following years. In truth, I remember all of them rather less vividly than the first. I remained (of course) in the fitness model and muscle model categories rather than bodybuilder and (equally of course) in the Masters or over-fifty age group. I trained hard for each of them and my nutrition was exactly where it should be, with very much the same dietary approach as I had for the first. But there was a key difference: for a couple of the contests, I experimented with taking additional sports supplements during the run up to the event as I described in Chapter 13. Nothing extreme, certainly nothing that would appear on a list of suspect substances.

Creatine and BCAAs were the main two supplements I tried, both for several weeks pre-event. These are two of the best-researched supplements in sports nutrition and are said, in combination, to contribute to muscle mass development and retention during dieting phases and to increasing endurance and to the reduction of fatigue. Finally, I also took a third supplement, the Ripped fat burner from Rob Riches' own company, True Performance Nutrition.

I can't remember which of the contests were the ones I used those supplements as preparation and, as I said in Chapter 13, I can't tell today by looking at the photos. In summary, I wasn't really sold on the supplement approach (as you'll know from that earlier chapter), and I haven't used any for the more recent contests.

One thing I did buy into was photoshoots, and I usually scheduled a shoot with Simon Howard as before or with Matt Marsh, another great fitness photographer, close to contest day on all my events. They used gym locations in London, Watford and High Wycombe, and the images from those days combine with the official photos and videos from the contests to make a great and very pictorial record of those times.

Back to St. Albans: Jenny was there to support me at every one of those contests and the actual few minutes on-stage was electrifying each time, just as it had been for the first, but I could feel that the appeal of Miami Pro had begun to drop. I picked up either a winner or runner-up trophy each time for both categories, but the moment when I thought: 'That was great, but I'm glad's it over' came more quickly with each passing event. The on-stage time remained a thrill, but the justification of the effort in the preparation phase for those joyous minutes became harder every time.

Eventually the organisers of Miami Pro decided to drop the over-fifties categories and make over-forties the new Masters. I can understand that as the number of competitors for the over-fifties was never great and I remember one year when there were just two of us. By then I was 58, so although I could present a stage-worthy physique with others over fifty, I wouldn't have been realistically comparable amongst athletes up to 18 years younger than me.

I made lots of friends at Miami Pro and wish them every success but five was enough. Any future Miami Pro events would be without me on the competitor list.

However, I still enjoyed the contest stage. I learned that Miami Pro is not the only organiser of these events, and entered contests with another federation, Pure Elite. I was interested to see how the approach of the two federations differed.

The two contests I undertook with Pure Elite, one in November 2014 and one in September 2015, were in the Beck Theatre in Hayes, near Heathrow. It was a nice change from St. Albans, but still not exactly exotic. Pure Elite's format was similar to Miami Pro in many ways. I was pleased to see Pure Elite didn't have the theme-wear rounds that Miami Pro had so I could leave my pilot's get up at home.

There was a Male Fitness Model over 45 category at Pure Elite. That would put me at 13 years older than the youngest allowable competitor, I could live with that much of an age difference. I remember there were more entrants than at Miami Pro; the reduction in five years meant a few additional entries in my age group.

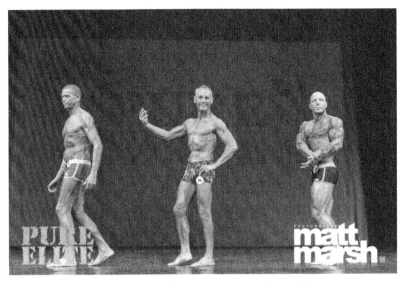

The top three of my age group at Pure Elite

As well as age groups, Pure Elite offered an interesting category called Body Transformation, in which the on-stage competitor would be judged against some 'before transformation' photos supplied by the entrant and projected on the large screen at the back of the stage.

The judges would score each competitor in the Body Transformation category by evaluating how impressive a body change had taken place. I supplied a few photos of the old obese version of me, and the change I had made obviously impressed the judges as, in the 2015 event, I came away with 4th place in a very large field drawn from every age group.

It was interesting to see that the transformations were about evenly split between obese-to-fit and scrawny-to-fit with a few entries of severely-ill-to-fit. Indeed, one of the severely-ill-to-fit entrants won.

Again, I made friends there amongst the competitors, two of whom, Nicola Chan and Rob Richley (not to be confused with Riches) will feature later in my story. But adding the two events from Pure Elite to the five from Miami Pro was enough.

After seven contests, I made the decision to hang up my stage trunks and bid farewell to the spray tan for good. I had a great time, collected trophies each time I competed, but now was the time to move on.

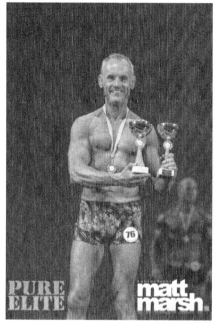
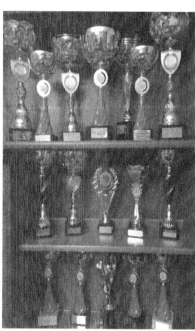

Collecting two trophies from Pure Elite   *The trophy cabinet at home*

So, I knew contests were behind me. What and where next? I wasn't heading for an out-of-shape destination. I wanted to expand my future as a fitness professional in new ways, some of which I had planned for, while I hoped others would arrive as surprise opportunities.

To do that I would have to spread the message about fitness, especially for the over fifties, by as many means as possible.

19 – Spreading the Word

I've been keen to spread the word to as many others as possible ever since I achieved my bodyfat loss, muscle gain and associated improvements in all my health and fitness measurements. I found much pleasure in this change and to use one of my favourite phrases again, I continue to believe that getting fit over fifty will add years to your life and life to those years. You may recall that I said that passing that message on to as many as I could is a fundamental aspect of my approach to helping others in my age group. Doing so forms part of the New Normal way of life for me.

It's not as altruistic as it sounds. I see myself as a fitness professional operating as a business and I attempt to make a modest profit from my commercially-focussed activities. However, my decisions are not governed by the need to generate a substantial income. If it's a fun versus profit decision on anything, then fun is likely to win. Secondly, to expand that fun comment, I am not going to do anything that I really don't enjoy doing. I'm at the stage of life that I don't need to do anything because I should, only because I choose to.

I know few people with that combination, in a position to being able to do what they want and not worry too much about the income. That's a key reason why I think that if anybody should be able to devote time and efforts to promoting fitness for this age group it should be me.

I've always been keen to receive enquiries from people of my age group interested in my approach and wanting to learn more. I am of course willing to help any genuine enquiry; but sometimes it can be more complicated and I've had many requests for an entire workout programme or nutrition plan. Some of my recommendations for these can be found on my website but a few years ago I felt that having some specific deliverables to offer to those interested would be a good approach. I created and documented a couple of workout systems[5] to meet this need: the first for people with limited time and a second, based very much on what I do myself, for those who can devote more time to fitness. This led to further standardised plans I created for nutrition and fitness-focussed recipe books[6].

I offer unlimited advice by email to anyone who purchases one of my courses and I like to follow up to see if my efforts have helped purchasers. I often hear: 'yes, Chris, I followed your course and my fitness has improved' and this is very gratifying. This proves that my message about the benefits of getting fitter in your fifties is not just being received but also being acted upon to reach a good conclusion, at least in some instances.

These days a key means of passing on messages is, of course, via social media. I'm not a fan of social media for personal use; one reason is that I've heard too many scary stories of what the tech giants do with all that data that people willingly supply to them relating to themselves, their friends, where they go, when they go, what they do, what they want to buy and their opinions on everything. I used to maintain personal Facebook and Twitter accounts, but I eventually realised I wasn't getting joy from using it, the opposite in fact, and combining that with my scepticism of the industry, I've used them less and less. My accounts are now close to dormant and I feel the happier for it.

On the other hand, I do believe in using social media channels to promote my fitness activity. I have a separate business Facebook account for Fitness Over Fifty and I have repurposed my Twitter account to be solely for my posts about fitness. I don't mind what those big corporations do with the data they extract from my messages on how to do exercises or my nutrition tips.

I discovered Instagram a few years ago. Again, I use it only for promoting my fitness activities and its image-centric messaging approach is ideal for information in a visual form, such as how to do an exercise, looking good on stage or in a photoshoot, or what a nutritionally balanced meal looks like. I've also discovered that I can post once to Instagram and the photo or video and text can automatically be copied to the Fitness Over Fifty Facebook page and my Twitter account, thus cutting down on social media input by me. It suits me perfectly that I can post to all three platforms just from a single entry on Instagram. These days that's all I do on those platforms, usually posting something once a week in that way. It doesn't take much of my time and it builds a base of people interested in what I do, some of whom go on to be my clients.

Another visually centred system I use is my Fitness over Fifty channel[7] on YouTube. I enjoy planning, recording, editing and posting fitness-related videos and receiving comments and reacting to them. There is a video library of all the exercises I recommend on my channel along with many examples of fitness activities with which I've been involved on stage, in gyms and elsewhere.

I was very surprised with the way YouTube took off for me. When I launched my first video, an Introduction to Fitness Over Fifty, featuring me on screen but actually filmed by Rob and his business partner Dmitry in Los Angeles, I expected it would eventually get maybe 100 views. I was stunned when it reached 1,000. Enthused by this response I started to create more videos and now, several years later, I'm close to half-a-million views in total of videos on my channel. There's a lot of enjoyable work gone into creating those videos and I hope that many views are people from my age group using the content to help increase their own fitness levels.

I've seen how many people come back to my YouTube Channel regularly. For many, it's not just a one-time visit, rather they want to watch and learn. Specifically for those who are like this, people who want a regular input of inspiration and education, I established a monthly subscription club[8] – Fit Club 50. Club members receive monthly newsletters including recipes, exercise tips, videos, infographics and articles and anything I can think of to go into a regular update and keep the recipients' interest levels up. I try to make Fit Club 50 as interactive as possible, encouraging fitness questions from members, which I always answer in subsequent editions. I encourage members to seek new joiners and in my first and only comparison with Brad Pitt I remind members to pass the message on: 'The first rule of Fit Club is: you do talk about Fit Club.'

Away from the printed word now and back to the visual medium. In 2013 I met Jason Gurr, an independent television content producer. He wanted to produce a one-hour TV documentary on an interesting person, spotted me online and asked if I would be willing to be the subject. You know me well enough by now to guess my reaction.

We started planning the programme. I sorted out filming locations and arranged for some of my fitness contacts to be available for on-screen interviews. After location work involving both of us and some editing, creating titles and adding music (all Jason's work), the documentary was ready. Jason had an agreement with The Community Channel to broadcast it and the programme was shown several times and viewable on Sky, Virgin and Freeview. Should you wish to see it now, there are no more repeats planned but it is on YouTube[9]. The name Jason and I came up with for the documentary was 'Fat to Fit at Fifty'. I liked the name so much I decided to keep it in mind for another project one day.

Let's move from vision-based communication to audio-based. You may recall that I enjoy radio presenting; I first mentioned that way back in Chapter 1 as something I did in my spare time at University. I still have that joy and have taken on a (very) part-time role as a presenter at community radio station MarlowFM 97.5. Based in the Buckinghamshire town in the station's name, the FM signal can be heard up to twenty miles away (including at the top of Heathrow Control Tower, where they really should be listening to other things, I feel). Thanks to broadcasts online and more recently apps like TuneIn Radio and smart-speaker systems like Alexa, the station can be heard worldwide.

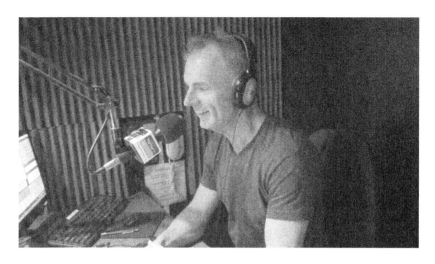

Spreading the word by radio - the MarlowFM studio

I presented a variety of shows for them for a couple of years. Then, a gap came up in the schedule on Tuesday mornings for a specialist health and fitness interview and discussion programme with some music too. A content mix rather like Jeremy Vine on BBC Radio 2 and with the same type of music. I filled that schedule slot and am still there today using the two hours to talk to guests, as well as passing on my own fitness thoughts from time to time. I try to arrange for two guests in every show. I've had yoga instructors, mental health specialists, nutritional therapists, personal trainers, osteopaths, charity fundraisers, trauma therapists and chefs, just to name the first few categories of guest that come to mind. Probably my most famous guest was locally based celebrity chef (and weight-loss success story) Tom Kerridge, who has been on my show a few times.

These days I'm one of a team who rotate as presenters for the show, with my turn coming around once or twice a month. The show is called Good Morning Marlow (Health and Fitness edition) and its still on Tuesday mornings. Feel free to listen[10], and if it is my turn to present, then phone-in or email a fitness question or a music request. I'll do my best to answer or play your selection.

One of my fellow presenters at the station was Chris Harper, a Media Studies student in his final year at Bucks New University in nearby High Wycombe. One day back in 2014 Chris mentioned to me that the University has a fully equipped TV studio on their campus, complete with editing suite and a mobile outside broadcast unit. That means all the facilities required to make broadcast-quality television programmes. One of the things that Chris mentioned is that the students in the final year on his course have to develop and undertake some practical TV programme production work and he was searching for a subject for his own project for this.

An idea was forming very quickly in my mind. With all the YouTube videos I had created, my interest in TV was growing. If I could supply programme ideas of interest, and all the content, would Chris and the University be willing to supply the technology and skills to record and edit it? A positive response from Chris and the University authorities suggested to me that this was to be a perfect match with winners on all sides. You can probably detect a lineage for my enthusiasm for this idea going straight back to Rob Riches.

I hooked up with a fitness friend, Keith Cormican, who agreed to be the co-presenter. We worked many late nights on the format and eventually we had the outline content for a series comprising four episodes of thirty minutes each. Keith was way under fifty, so we decided to make this a magazine-format series of fitness programmes suitable for all ages rather than just for my over-fifties area of specialisation. I came up with the title 'Fit Happens', as the name appealed to me and it rhymes with, well, something I'm sure.

That first series of four episodes took two days of in-studio filming, and a similar time of filming on location - all near home. Chris Harper was the cameraman, producer and editor, pulling in other students from the Media Studies faculty as required for additional tasks involved in the production.

If I say so myself, the four episodes were quite impressive, especially when it is remembered that all the on-screen people were amateurs in TV, and all the behind-the-scenes folk were students. And produced on a budget of zero (OK, I did buy some food on location and some beers – so make that £30 budget in total).

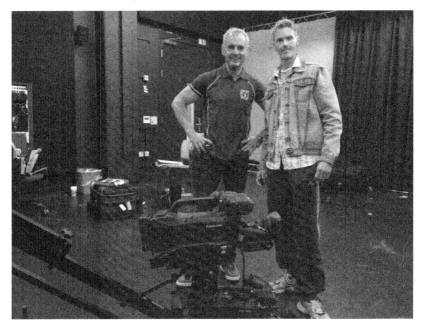

With Keith in the Bucks New University studio for Fit Happens Series One

I had retained some contacts at The Community Channel following on from the earlier documentary and asked if they would be interested in showing the series. They agreed. That was the one thing of course that Chris and the University couldn't do. Record, edit, sound engineer, graphics – yes, they could do all that; but actually broadcast it, no. Legal documents were drawn up giving the Channel the right to broadcast and as with the earlier documentary, each episode of Fit Happens was shown several times over the course of a few months in 2014 and 2015.

Move on a year and Chris Harper had graduated with Fit Happens as part of his degree submission. Then the idea of a second series of Fit Happens came up. A new generation of students were in the same position that Chris had been in earlier, looking for a subject and for some content upon which to create a TV programme for their own final-year degree submissions. Somehow resisting the temptation to call it 'Fit Happens – The Next Generation', the idea for the second series was born.

I discussed the project with the head student on this new production, Charles Battison, and jointly we decided to make the second series bigger, bolder and brighter than the first. We used a much larger pool of students in the technical team, newer technologies (you've never seen so much green screen), better locations and the biggest enhancement of all, a third presenter alongside Keith and me. The new host was Nicola Chan, who I had met at the Pure Elite contest as she was also a competitor at that event.

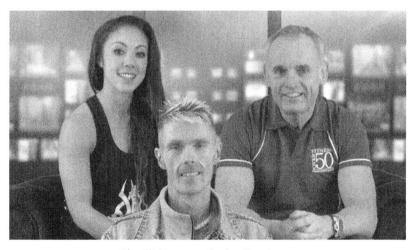

The Fit Happens Series Two team

Nicola enhanced the show massively, bringing her own skills, wit and personality with her. With new graphics and with the series now extended to five episodes, Series Two of Fit Happens excelled Series One in every respect and with the same limitations as the first series: everyone amateurs and students. With a bigger crew, the budget went up – probably up to around £150 if I included all the beer and sandwiches. The Community Channel showed it from 2017 and still retains the rights to do so in the Channel's new guise of Together TV. It has spread geographically too, as the series has been supplied by the Channel to community-based TV stations around the world including

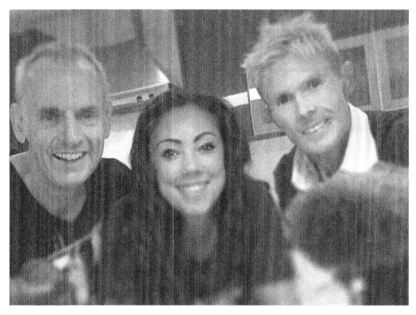

On-set in the kitchen

America's PBS. The most recent data suggests that perhaps around a million people have viewed at least one of the episodes.

It was hard work but very enjoyable and the two series of the Fit Happens TV series[11] are something of which everyone who was involved can be extremely proud. Where is everyone now? Chris and Charles both have successful careers in broadcast media, as do many of the other members of the crew. Nicola is a fitness professional with her own large group of enthusiastic clients and also hosts a show on a local radio station in West London called HayesFM.

Keith sadly passed away, losing a battle with cancer that he had kept secret from everyone on the series. I know he was happy with the work he had contributed on development and production and in hosting both series. Those two series of the Fit Happens TV programme are a legacy that all those that knew Keith can still view.

Will there be a third series of Fit Happens? Surely there's another generation of Media Studies students available to take over now that Charles has followed Chris out of university and into professional video work. I decided not to do that, partially because it didn't seem right without Keith; and whatever we did it would have been hard to top the quality of Series Two. At the back of my mind, when seeing the finished second series, I did wonder if the idea might be taken up by one of the big TV channels in the UK. In my moments of unjustified optimism, I saw the third series as being a Top Gear but for fitness. Imagine where we could have gone and what we could have done with some real budgets allocated to it by a national channel. I tried, as did Charles, to interest the major UK networks in the idea but nobody took it up.

So, after two series I decided to pull the plug on Fit Happens as an idea for a third TV series. I had registered the name in the UK and I still use it. One of my delivered fitness courses bears the name and I have also started a podcast series[12], 'The Fit Happens Podcast', which comprises mainly chats with people that I originally interviewed on MarlowFM.

Actually, it wasn't quite the end of 'Fit Happens' on TV, since there were two further outings for the name on the small screen. They involve me and a gentleman that I will introduce to you in the next chapter.

20 – Paying it Forward

You will have read quite a few times by now that I see it as a key part of my life these days to pass on the message of the benefits of getting fit at any age to as many people as I can. It has made such a difference to me and I want as many others as possible to see my story as an inspiration for changes they can make to their own lives.

Every time you've read that message so far, I have been thinking of the audience being in the same age group as me or older – in their fifties or above. However, a few years ago I had the chance to move in the opposite direction and apply that same philosophy to someone far younger than me. Doing so led to a renewed interest in some fitness activities for which I had begun to lose enthusiasm; and indeed, moved my life on as a fitness professional to create and take a few entirely new opportunities.

How did this happen? Let me set the scene.

There is an annual event at the NEC in Birmingham called Bodypower. Usually held over four days of a May Bank Holiday weekend, it is the top expo for the fitness industry. There is a major emphasis on the physique side – it's the number one show for bodybuilders, strength athletes and fitness models in the UK. Just about everyone involved at any level in those three fields in the UK is present.

On the exhibitor side the three biggest categories are companies that provide supplements, weights and equipment, and fitness apparel. They know it's the one place that they can interface directly with members of their target market in person, where they can show their latest offerings with the maximum chance of influencing sales and indeed, where their sponsored athletes can present to their likely customers and be ready for selfies with expo attendees on their stands. Those attending Bodypower as individuals want to be successful in any of the three target fields, all hoping to buy the items they need, to meet the influencers and their hero athletes and to learn whatever they can to increase their chances of success, enjoyment and perhaps employment within their chosen specialisation in fitness.

It's a massive event that grows bigger and better every year. If you have not been, you would be stunned to see how large an event it is with hundreds of companies present on stands and thousands of people attending each day. As most folk in this industry are younger than me, I'm never surprised to see only a small number of people in my age group amongst the crowds; but the word must be getting out because last year there was a dedicated zone for Over Fifties Fitness, where I had been invited to make a few presentations. It wasn't the busiest part of the expo floor but I think I had around eighty people to one of my seminars, which was gratifying. But I'm getting ahead of myself, so let's go back eight years to the first year I attended, 2012.

Rob Riches used to attend Bodypower annually with a stand devoted to his supplement and clothing company, True Performance Nutrition. He would come back from the USA for the event with his girlfriend and would ask her, me and others he knew in the UK to help out on the stand. Often Rob would be chatting to his fans amongst the show attendees and agreeing to appear in their selfies, so it was left to the rest of us to man the shop, so to speak. It wasn't tough work and there was plenty of free time to wander around the expo, meet old friends and develop new contacts. For example, it was while doing this that I met Keith Cormican, later to join me on the sofas in the Fit Happens TV studio.

After two years of this I felt like a change, as did Rob. So, for 2014 he didn't have a stand but instead asked me (and a few others) to walk around the exhibition floor wearing a t-shirt from his company, chatting to people and just being friendly. This was the month after I had competed in the Miami Pro World Championships again and picked up first place in Muscle Model Over Fifty category. By that time, I was very used to competing with the Miami Pro organisation, and I had decided to move on, since the trophy cupboard at home was getting nicely full and it was time to close the Miami Pro competing chapter of my life. If you've read the book this far, you will know that wasn't quite what happened, and here's why.

It was while walking the floor at Bodypower expo that year that a young guy came up to me, pointed at my branded t-shirt and said – 'True Performance Nutrition, that's Rob Riches' company isn't it?' Having confirmed that it was, we started to chat. And we didn't stop, for an hour or more.

That was my introduction to Dan Wynes and also his rather patient girlfriend, who was good at listening to us talk fitness for that hour. It turned out that Dan was a former GB-team standard schoolboy for gymnastics, and since he is 35 years younger than me, those school days were very recent for him. He was looking for a new challenge in life, had discovered the weights area at his local gym, had heard others there talking about Bodypower, did some research and came along to see what all the fuss was about. I passed on many of my thoughts on training, nutrition and the lifestyle factors affecting fitness; and Dan listened well. One thing about people in their early twenties is that if they are sufficiently interested – and Dan was – they learn very quickly, a bit of a contrast with my own rather less rapid brain these days.

Dan said that he wanted to make fitness into both a hobby and a career. Towards the end of our conversation, we discussed whether we should form some kind of mentoring relationship, whereby I would give advice and suggestions to Dan on helping him achieve success in this new direction. I wasn't entirely sure I knew what was expected of me as a mentor – something less than a coach or trainer, something more than sending out blogs and info. Anyway, he said three things that made me inclined to accept, and a fourth that sealed the deal.

The three things were that (a) following his earlier research into the fitness industry he was a fan of Rob Riches and his company True Performance Nutrition; (b) he thought that things I had accomplished in the fitness world – the contests, the TV show, the PT business – were great (flattery gets you everywhere with me); and (c) his girlfriend was very keen to see him progress to reach his goals. The fourth was that when I questioned him about perhaps training with a deadline of a competition for him, his eyes lit up and the enthusiasm flowed from him. I was convinced to work with him as his mentor.

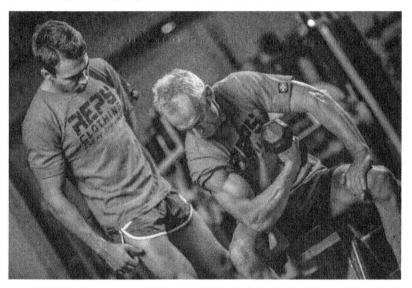

Practical mentoring in the gym

Dan and I communicated most days, discussing obvious areas such as training and nutrition, but also topics such as stage presence and posing for the contest, workout planning and recording, social media positioning, creating YouTube content, photo and video shoots, self-promotion and publicity. Although I wouldn't claim to be an expert, these are all areas in which I have gathered some experience over the years.

We visited each other many times in the months that followed, despite the 120 miles distance between our homes, either by his coming south or by my heading to his home in Shropshire. A visit either way would always be for gym workouts of course, and taking progress photos and contributing to the growing mass of documentation. And Dan's progress was nothing short of phenomenal, which was a result of 1% of my input, and 99% of what I call ABCDE on his (that's Absolute Bloody-minded Commitment, Determination and Effort). I've never seen anyone train as hard or as consistently or be as perfect in adhering to nutrition rules or as determined to be a success. He very quickly became qualified as a Personal Trainer and my views on the work ethic of the generation younger than mine were being rewritten, at least in this one example.

I've learned that the mentor gets as much from the mentoring relationship as the mentee. The time I spent with Dan reinvigorated my own training, so much so that I decided to drop all this nonsense about retiring from contests and to enter the same contest as Dan, the Pure Elite in November that year. Because the training and up-coming contest world was all so new to him, he saw it through fresh eyes and this refreshed my outlook too. Dan had asked me to mentor him so I could pass information and tips to him. Little did either of us realise that I would benefit at least as much from the passion and energy flowing in the opposite direction.

A couple of months before the show date Dan and I decided we would go to LA for a week of intense training coming back just a few days before the contest itself. We had the approval of both Jenny and Dan's girlfriend for our trip, and both of them were already looking forward to seeing us on stage back in the UK. The plans Dan and I developed for that week would have me training like the 21-year-old that I was with, and that led to an idea.

Perhaps this story of mentorship and friendship across the generations would be of interest to other people in the UK? Having had the Fit Happens series on TV, was there now room for a one-off special focussing on Dan and me and our training for the contest? I discussed those two questions with The Community Channel. Their response was yes to both and as a result the idea for a one-off special was launched. I already had a friendly editor to work with in the UK and Rob put me in touch with a student cameraman in California. The opening shots of the show would be Dan issuing me a challenge to be 'the best of your generation' in the upcoming contest, and me issuing exactly the same challenge to him. Those two scenes inspired the name of the special – Fit Happens: Generation Challenge.[13]

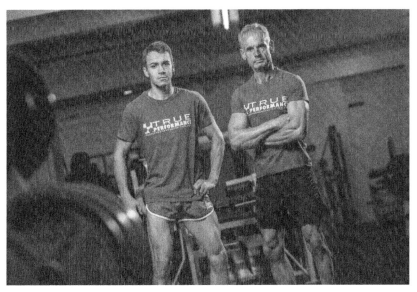

Preparing for the Fit Happens: Generation Challenge

Over in California that student cameraman followed me and Dan for a full day, recording while we did our dawn cardio running up and down the famous Santa Monica stairs, breakfasting in the rented apartment, working out at Gold's gym and taking advantage of the setting California sunshine with a second workout in the open air at Muscle Beach. By the end of that day and that week, we were exhausted but happy. We were as ready as we were going to be for the contest and had recorded some great footage. We said goodbye to the blue Pacific Ocean and looked forward to our next trip to the seaside.

This was to the rather less blue Thames Estuary at Margate, the venue for the Pure Elite Fitness Model Championships in November 2014. I was doing what I had supposedly retired from – just this once, just to help Dan; nothing to do with my enjoying some more stage time, of course.

Naturally, Dan and I were in separate age groups, he was in the Juniors (under 25) and I the Masters (over 45). Both of our good ladies cheered like mad whenever either of their two spray-tanned grinning chaps were on stage and, looking back in the day, we were both happy with our performances. The conclusion was that we had some further footage from our stage appearances to conclude the Fit Happens: Generation Challenge special and, well, one of us had a trophy.

I picked up 3rd place in a field of six entrants, and sadly Dan came home empty-handed. I had no doubt that he was in the best shape of his life so far, but there were around 30 people in his age group, meaning his was a much tougher category for him than mine was for me. It was another trophy for me and a good time to call a halt to my competing.

That was until (oh no) I changed my mind again. Of course, Dan wasn't happy with being less than the best at Margate, especially with TV cameras there, and a contest victory was in his mind an essential step in his career. He had recently decided to pursue a career as a fitness model contest coach and a winner's trophy would look good on his CV and newly-developed website.[14]

So, two years later we were doing the same all over again. Back to LA for a week of dedicated training with filming for a final outing for the Fit Happens TV brand. This time it was Fit Happens: Generation Revenge[15]. Back home and it was a day-return to St. Albans for the fifth (and final, really) time for me on the Miami Pro stage. But this time Dan won his category in the recently created Mr Model class, which had a huge trophy. I think it's his proudest possession; and so it should be for the amount of work that over the years he put into winning it.

The titles of those two TV specials, Generation Challenge and Generation Revenge, may make it sound as though Dan and I were against one another, trying to come ahead of the other in a competitive situation. I suppose that positioning may have attracted viewers to the TV shows but it was far from the truth. In reality we both wanted each of us to do well. We were in separate age classifications in the contests so we could both have come first. There would be competition from others sharing the same stage but none between us.

Let's move forward another year. It's now 2017, Dan and I remain good friends and the supply of ideas and suggestions flows in both directions. Indeed, it hadn't been a one-way mentoring for years. I had eight contests behind me (five Miami Pro, three Pure Elite) and I didn't feel like any more. I had definitely retired from the contest stage (again).

Then I unretired (again). Maybe I should retire from retiring. I had definitely had my fill of the contest stage in the UK. But I had noticed contests in the US, specifically some that take place three times a year at Muscle Beach. Being a fan of the fitness scene in Southern California, I decided to enter one: The Muscle Beach Championships of September 2017. By this time, Dan was a successful coach with a string of clients (mainly female) who were winning trophies at events in the UK; and one thing in fitness that Dan and I hadn't tried together was some formal pre-contest coaching.

I agreed with Dan that he would be my coach for the final couple of months up to contest time. The fact that Dan still lived in Shropshire was not a problem, since most of his coaching clients maintain their relationship with him online. And the fact that we were long-term friends as well as coach/trainee did not mean that I was in for an easy ride from his coaching routines. Not an exercise was undertaken and rarely did a calorie pass my lips in the final few weeks that Dan didn't know about, or indeed instruct. He demands nothing less than the

161

100% ABCDE (see above) from himself, and isn't interested in clients that don't do the same.

The natural end to that was a week in Los Angeles, the third and last one that Dan and I undertook together. No cameras this time. I think we had developed the Generation Challenge/Revenge concept as far as we could. And Dan wasn't competing; he was coaching and wanted to concentrate on that role. Firstly, he designed the plans for my training three times a day. Dan performed his own workouts too and he didn't have to watch every set and rep I did, as he trusted me to do that. He also cooked and controlled everything I ate in that final week. I will admit to cheating once on some homemade banana bread once that week but Dan found out. I was the naughty schoolboy and he was justly annoyed by it. I could be trusted in the gym but not in the kitchen, he concluded. Sorry, who is the sixty-year-old and who is 24 here?

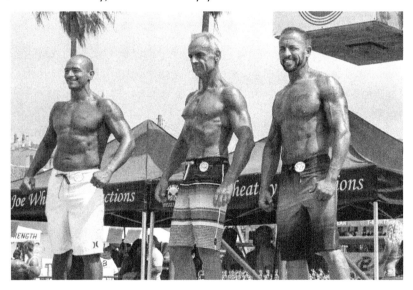

On stage at Muscle Beach

The week ended with the contest stage for me, entered into the two senior age-group categories, the over 45s and over 35s for Physique, the American term for what the UK calls Fitness Modelling. I entered both, without much of a hope in the 35s, but I replayed a thought from my very first contest days: if I was going through that much preparation, I might as well go for ten minutes on stage rather than five. So, the Over 35s as well as the Over 45s, both in the Physique category, it was to be.

It was very different to a Pure Elite or Miami Pro. To start with it was in the open air, luckily in glorious September sunshine. Another difference was that before going on stage competitors could warm-up in the open-air gym behind the stage; that was somewhere that I had trained, with and without Dan, on many occasions in the past. Also, spectators could come and go as they pleased. There is banked seating ('bleachers' is the American term) for around 500 spectators with no admission fee. And finally, it was the first fitness contest I had entered without Jenny rooting for me.

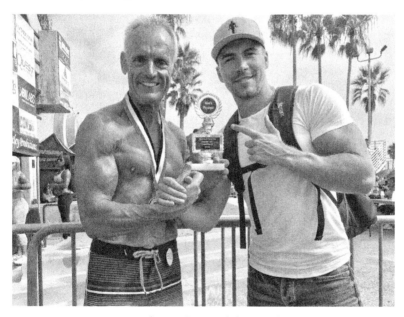

The student with his coach

I picked up a fifth-place trophy in one of the categories which made it all worthwhile. I was way over the age of most of the competitors and despite Dan driving me to being probably in the best shape of my life I hadn't really expected to win anything. I was happy for myself but also for Dan. He now had another client with a trophy for his own coaching track record; and I had concluded my contest career with an event at Muscle Beach, the spiritual home of physique and bodybuilding. Eight contests in the UK and a final one in California. Nice.

Dan and I still see each other, not as often as in the past, but we are both willing to swap ideas with each other whenever we can. He has gone on to further success, arranging and promoting his own contests and most recently taking up a contract with the Bodypower organisation for two years in India, travelling around the country raising the profile of fitness modelling, physique competitions and the Bodypower branded gyms that he is helping to launch. I've no idea where that will eventually take him but I'm sure he will be dedicated to a level unknown by most. Jenny has come up with a term for Dan based on his commitment and approach: 'the youngest middle-aged person I know' – which is, I assure you, a compliment, not an insult!

To bring this part of the story to a close I'm going back to the first of those three trips for Dan and me to California. One evening Rob Riches invited us to dinner at the house he shares with his girlfriend. At one point when she and Dan were out of the room, Rob turned to me and said words to the effect that he thinks it's great the way that I am passing on to Dan my love of fitness, the enthusiasm to go the extra mile, and a willingness to create new opportunities. He felt he had passed these on to me and now he saw me passing them on again. He knew that I did that with those of the same age or older than me, and now here I was doing the same with someone much younger.

Paying it forward was the term he used. He thought it a very good thing to do.

21 – Was it a Good Time?

You have read that gym training is my number one fitness activity. The combination of those afternoon or evening gym visits with my morning cardio, plus some stretching and abs later in the day, forms my normal daily routine. Those were the activities that took me from fat to fit a decade ago.

For the first four or so years of my fitness journey that routine described my exercise life. But that changed around 2010 and since then I have tried a few other sports, some of which have become almost as much a part of my life as going to the gym. Almost.

There were three reasons for adding these additional activities to my life. Firstly, it's the joy of doing something that I couldn't have done earlier. Without exception my old obese self could not have achieved any of the activities I am going to describe. I simply didn't have the strength or stamina and I had too much weight to move. Losing that excess bodyfat and adding some muscle enabled me not just to do these new things but to enjoy doing them too.

Secondly, I was keen to build more time with Jenny into my life. All the sports and events I am now going to describe are those that Jenny regularly took part in and were important to her. Yes, we went to the gym together occasionally and she was enthusiastic about my physique competitions and everything else I did in fitness, but all of that was activity by me and both of us wanted to increase our time spent as a couple. Of course, we spent many hours a week together, going out, watching TV, visiting friends and so on, but next to no time doing anything sports or exercise-focussed together. This was a bit nuts now I think about it, as we both loved our own fitness events; but in the main they were separate activities, enjoyed massively, but enjoyed separately.

Finally, all these new sports and activities would add to my fitness levels. It's not as though I was adding something that would detract from progress or dropping something positive already undertaken. They would all contribute to both halves of my philosophy of adding years to my life, and life to my years.

So, what were Jenny's sports that I could perhaps add to my own activity list? The big three for her were swimming, cycling and running plus putting those three together into a fourth sport, triathlon. Jenny has plenty of medals and trophies from her success, probably the highlight being a couple of Ironman-distance triathlons in which she has taken part. Both of those demanded 12 hours of continuous effort from her. Well, I'm not up for the Ironman distances nor for that length of time, but I'll give a shorter course triathlon a go and also the three individual sports, especially if I'm doing them with Jenny.

I may as well start at the bottom, which I where I would probably be heading in most swimming pools. Swimming is one thing that I've always been particularly poor at, and even adding those years of changing from doing zero exercise to doing lots I still don't enjoy swimming. Yes, I love playing around in a pool and in the sea (especially if the sea is warm, a nice shade of blue and a long flight from home) but swimming in a way calculated to cover a distance in as short a time as possible is not for me. Yes, I know I now have the strength and stamina and I'm sure my technique would become a thousand percent better with some lessons, but I just don't enjoy it. Let's move on; I would have to accompany Jenny on other sports.

Cycling is a good next stop. Like just about every schoolkid, I cycled a lot in my early years. Going out with friends after school (or sometimes when we should have been in school) would be a cycle trip, sometimes a whole day out, and my parents didn't worry. Life was gentler in the 1960's. But by the time I was at University, I didn't cycle at all; I didn't even own a bike. I can't put a date on it, but I probably invested in one about the age of 52 and started joining Jenny on a few leisure rides around home and maybe for day rides if we are away on holiday somewhere.

One of the benefits of cycling for me is that it is a great way to visit interesting pubs. As you know I'm enthusiastic on traditional ale and the pubs that serve them. Now I can add enthusiasm in the means of transport to and from them as well. Jenny and I started by setting as our first destination one of the pubs I love, which is a couple of miles away across fields and through woodland, twice as far by road. Soon we were expanding our cycle-pub trips, and trips of up to around twenty miles were soon on the agenda. Of course, a pub visit is never going to be a health-focussed activity, but if I am going to go, it's certainly healthier to cycle than drive.

I upgraded my ownership of bikes by two by adding a mountain bike and a road bike to the all-purpose bike I had (which I now know is called a hybrid). In my younger days the road bike was known as a racer but it must have been renamed during my non-cycling years. Jenny has said that the number of bikes you need is n+1, where n is the number of bikes you already own. That sounds like a good theory to me and I have adhered to it by replacing two of the bikes over the years without actually disposing of the previous ones. I like to have a spare or two in case we have visitors that we can persuade into a pub ride.

Going beyond the pub trips, we have ridden many longer distance routes and the occasional event. I have a particular liking for cycling on old scenic railway routes (maybe because of the lack of hills) and Jenny and I have embarked on such trips ranging from Cornwall to the Highlands. Another type of ride I particularly like is to ride one way on a preserved railway by train and cycle back across country keeping near the line for a view of any steam trains on the way. The Severn Valley and North Yorkshire Moors are probably my favourite such heritage railway-and-bike rides.

You can perhaps tell that I became enthusiastic about cycling. It is a means of transportation, a way of seeing places and getting closer to them in a way you can't in a car, and it's also a means of exercise. What isn't cycling for me? It's never been a competitive sport; I've never been in a race where I am alongside other riders with the objective of trying to beat them. I do try for a decent result when I'm being timed but it's always my time against my previous time and never me against that cyclist over there. Perhaps I could push it harder than I do but I always prioritise enjoyment over beating a time.

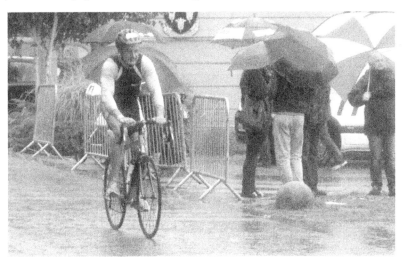

Not the happiest I have been on a bike, to be honest

An example of that was when Jenny and I did the Prudential Ride London Surrey 100 with 60,000 others. It is a timed event, but I was interested only in enjoying myself and taking in the views; and my only concern on timing was being at the finish in The Mall before the cut-off time, to avoid not being counted as a finisher. It was an interesting ride to say the least. The start was from the Queen Elizabeth Olympic Park in Stratford and the first few miles went well, then the heavens opened with rainfall as I have rarely seen it. Halfway through Richmond Park the ride was halted for twenty minutes due to flooding. Later on, as the ride entered Surrey and the rain continued to fall, the organisers removed the two steepest sections of the route, Leith Hill and Box Hill, declaring them to be too dangerous. The 100-mile route had been shortened to become a Ride 86.

Even as the rain eased there was still flooding to contend with. There is a section of road between Esher and Kingston where the road goes through a tunnel under railway tracks. I know the road but never seen in one foot deep in water before. Some tried to cycle, others walked their bikes; everyone was soaked.

Not a day for a getting a good time, but Jenny and I succeeded in being at the finish within the allotted time. We had a lift arranged from a friend to take us home from Trafalgar Square. I think he's forgiven us for the amount of water we left on his seats and in the footwells.

Another timed cycling event that Jenny and I did together was one where rain definitely wasn't a concern. This was the Cape Argus ride, which includes cycling from the Indian Ocean to the Atlantic. Actually, that is not quite as far as it sounds. It takes place in Cape Town and south of that city, so the part crossing between oceans is only about 10km of the overall 108km route.

It is said to be the most beautiful cycle race in the world (said by the organisers, that is) and it incorporates three very stiff climbs. Notable amongst these is Chapman's Peak, a 5km continuous climb with gradients up to 7%, where the riders cycle northbound with the Atlantic on their left on the way back into the city.

The organisers are correct in their description. The views are indeed stunning, assuming you have the energy to turn your head a little bit to the left to see them.

Shortly after Chapman's the riders encounter Suikerbossie. Despite the translation, there is nothing sweet about this hill. It's a long climb with gradients up to 8% and inland, so no sea views here. Many of the cyclists had given up at this point, given up riding that is, walking their bikes instead; but I kept going in (or usually just above) the saddle. Never have I needed the lowest gearing quite so much on a road bike.

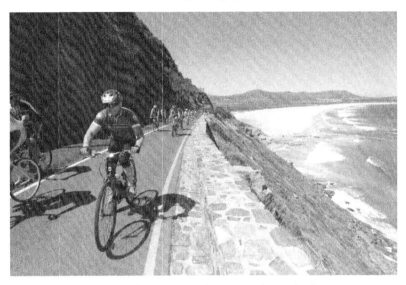

Chapman's Peak - much steeper than it looks

Although parts of the ride are in urban areas there are many rural parts with their own unique hazards. One of these is baboon activity; they like to jump on to the backs of riders from overhanging trees. Apparently, they also like sipping the remains of the high-carb energy gels that some riders ahead will have used and discarded, so now you have crazed baboons on a sugar rush leaping onto you. That's not something I worried about in Richmond Park, even with the soggy deer.

There's one other ride I want to mention and this was a sponsored ride I undertook for the Royal British Legion from London to Brussels with overnight stops in Calais and Ypres. The latter is of course famous for its role in commemorating the losses of life in the First World War and a place of massive significance to the charity. Jenny wasn't on this one, but my friends John, Jeremy and Tom cycled with me and, calling ourselves 'Les Poulets', you can see we weren't expecting to produce impressive performances. The first eighty miles were incredibly easy.

Due to some last-minute administrative problem, there was no agreement with the authorities for this ride to operate on public roads in the UK, so all the riders travelled in comfort by Eurostar to Calais while the bikes went in the backs of the ride-support road vehicles.

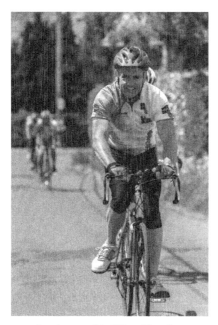

On the road in West Flanders

The next two days were, unsurprisingly, rather tougher. For these sections, totalling 200km, the cyclists were accompanied by motorcycle outriders who went ahead and blocked the side roads from joining traffic while the cycles crossed the junctions. For this reason, the riders had to stay in a fairly close group and the distance from the front to the rear of the group was probably around 400 metres. This required us to keep up with the group, which might have been a problem had there been a keen rider up front and one of us Chickens at the back.

To marshal the riders there was a lead car going at a moderately sedate pace with an illuminated 'Ne dépassez pas!' sign, so that controlled the front end. And at the rear, any laggards were picked up with their bikes by one of the support vehicles which then whizzed past the peloton and deposited the rider and bike a good distance in front even of the lead car. I took advantage of that once when my laggard's pace had got the better of me, being combined with a bout of hay fever as well as some fairly ferocious Flemish cobblestones.

We arrived ceremonially in Brussels where the Chickens consumed various Trappist ales and the charity benefitted from a hefty cheque.

As you see cycling is back into my life in a big way after a gap of getting on for fifty years. Now I want to move to two legs rather than two wheels and get activities with Jenny back into the story.

You will have read back in Chapter 11 that my fitness routine has included pre-breakfast cardio since the earliest days of my conversion to fitness. Originally that was solely on a cross-trainer but eventually I alternated that with treadmill running. Why had this change taken place? Because I had become a runner. That is a word that anyone knowing me at age 49 or before would find hard to apply to me. My level of obesity as well as my year of Achilles Tendon injury made that clear. As you know the bodyfat went away, the Achilles Tendon recovered and running came into my life.

Jenny had been a runner for as long as I can remember and is a keen member of the local running club. She had hoped for years to urge me into running both for fitness and for the sake of doing things together and eventually it happened. It wasn't a 'Couch to 5k' course for me (they didn't exist in those days) but a little thing called parkrun (which always has a lower case 'p' at the front and who am I to change that?). It is an event that takes place every week at hundreds of locations around the world, always on a Saturday, and in most countries at 9am. Despite the name not all locations are in parks and you don't have to run. In fact, you are encouraged to participate even if you can't run a single metre of the 5km distance. That tempted me, that and the fact that Jenny had been running in our local parkrun at Black Park in Slough most weeks for the previous year or so. We saw this as potentially a good way to increase our time together.

I registered and on Saturday, 5 June 2010 I attempted my first parkrun. Not just my first parkrun but also my first time ever running anything like 5km. I have a dim memory of being forced to run 400m around a track on a school sports day, but I don't think I ran a longer distance until that June day almost half a century later.

I had lost my excess bodyfat and put on some muscle by that stage. It was after my Year of Fitness and just checking my spreadsheet now shows that I was at the target numbers – 11 stone 7 pounds (161lb, 73kg) at 14.6% bodyfat. Those figures made me think I might not be totally rubbish at this; and what's more there were guys taking part who looked a lot less fit than me and if they could do it, maybe I could. Despite this as Jenny and I mingled with the starting group of runners, I wasn't confident and the 5km finish line seemed very far away. I formulated my strategy: to start off doing a bit of a run, see how far I could go, then walk while I got my breath back, then repeat. It was a massive reassurance to me that this wasn't a race so I wasn't in competition with anyone, not even myself this time as I hadn't ever run anything like this distance before.

I surprised myself massively in three ways: firstly, I was still on that initial run when I crossed the finish line without ever having slowed to a walk. Secondly, I really enjoyed it. I had recorded a time of just over 27 minutes and was smiling. Jenny was so glad to see me happy at the finish line and with her year of parkrun experience before me, she knew before I did that parkrun would become a big part of our lives together from that point on. I also noticed how I wasn't the only one smiling. The mental health benefits of this activity were beginning to dawn on me.

Nearly ten years later I have run parkrun over 300 times, nearly all with Jenny, although she had a serious injury which has kept her away from running in recent years. We have travelled the world with parkrun as our usual companion in every country and city, undertaking parkruns on most continents as well as all over the UK. We never plan a holiday or a weekend away without checking the location of the nearest parkrun for our regular Saturday morning fix, even if Jenny has been a spectator for a few years and may be for some time to come.

My favourite parkrun location was probably San Francisco, running at the waterside under the Golden Gate. Although rather less famous as a location, our local parkrun in Black Park in Slough is a beautiful one especially on a sunny morning with its tall pine trees. I think I know

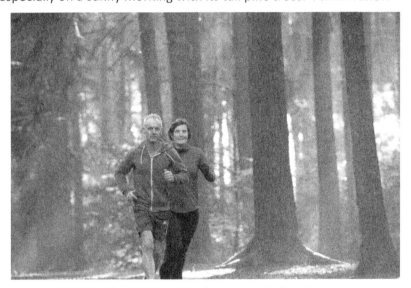

A favourite parkrun location - Black Park

each tree individually by now as I've run the course on over 200 occasions, often running as pacer for those who want a particular time.

Jenny and I would love to do some parkruns in Japan, and perhaps we will do once she has recovered. I would also love to run the parkrun in Yakutsk in Siberia, as I believe it's the furthest drive or rail trip from any other parkrun on the planet. I suspect we won't ever do that one.

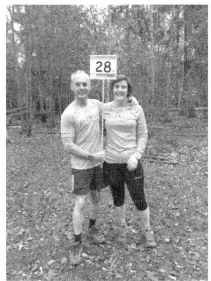 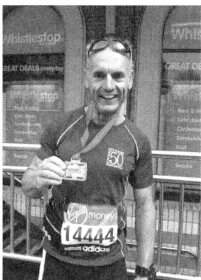

Pacing at Black Park parkrun   *Completing London Marathon*

Jenny and I have tried a few longer distances, I've now finished seven marathons and Jenny a total of nineteen. It was a thrill to do a marathon in my home city of London, passing so many locations I knew well from my days of commuting to the City. I was surprised by how many spectators in the Isle of Dogs somehow knew my first name and cheered me on, which helped during a tough part of the course. How come they knew me? I found out that I had spent almost the whole loop of the Island running next to someone who had his first name boldly printed on the front of his shirt. Whoever he was, I hope Chris didn't mind my absorbing some of the goodwill targeted at him.

My capability isn't up to tackling the full 26-mile marathon distance by running all the way. The strategy that has usually worked for me is to run the first 5k (I know I can do that now) then break the remainder into time blocks, typically periods of eight minutes running, two minutes walking – and that gets me around a marathon in about five hours.

As you know, I'm more interested in enjoying the event than setting a new time. Five hours will do nicely.

Except on one particular marathon. It's the one I would be really upset for completing in five hours. Actually, I want to take over six and ideally as close to six hours, thirty minutes as possible. It's the only marathon I've entered more than once, and indeed Jenny and I have run it together three times. And each year we crossed the finish line within the final 15 minutes before that six-and-a-half-hour cut-off time.

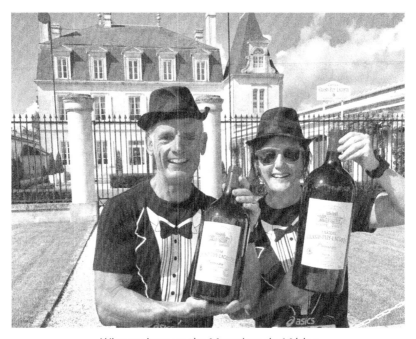

Wine waiters on the Marathon du Médoc

This is the Marathon du Médoc, a run which links together more than twenty of the finest wine chateaux in Médoc near Bordeaux on its 26-mile route. Many of these chateaux have live music, most are in stunning locations and all of them provide their own production for consumption by the runners during the event. Now that makes a change from the refreshment stops on most long runs. You're unlikely to see Chateau Lafitte Rothschild getting poured into rows of glasses by the gallon anywhere else. I'm sure that the chateaux aren't putting their very best vintages out for thirsty runners but, even so, it's a big upgrade from a plastic cup of water. There are also goodies such as oysters and steak to be had at the refreshment stops, alongside the more usual marathon event fare, such as bananas if you insist.

Not many people take the event totally seriously, 90% run in fancy dress (including us), and the real incentive to run more quickly on each leg is in order to spend more time at the next lovely chateau. It's known as the longest marathon in the world as the average time taken by runners is longer than other marathons; and I think I know why. By the way, I'm not going to claim that the wine added anything to the fitness benefits of running those 26 miles in the South West France sunshine, and I wouldn't recommend it more than once a year. But for that once per annum, well, it makes for an enjoyable and memorable occasion.

So, I'm a runner and a cyclist. I tried following in Jenny's footprints and entered a couple of triathlons, but the initial swimming leg on both of them dissuaded me from doing any more. Being close to people in the water who are determined to do well, sometimes getting their hands or feet in my face as they pushed hard, did nothing for me except to reinforce my acknowledged lack of ability in the skills required for that first leg. I could not see myself ever enjoying it, so I will be sticking to the cycling and running.

Reviewing this chapter brings a few conclusions to my mind. One is restating what I said at the beginning. Every activity I've mentioned would have been impossible for me to accomplish at age fifty or before. Partaking in these has brought Jenny and me ever closer together and enabled us to see parts of the world we wouldn't otherwise have visited. Jenny has had several operations to help the repair and recovery from her injury and I have no doubt that, one day, she will be back running and cycling better than ever. And we'll be doing it together again.

There is one real notable difference between my time in the gym and my doing the other sports I've described here. I started keeping gym records back at the year dot and I keep track of my recent numbers on the morning cardio; but not for running or cycling events. Since I prioritise enjoyment over results and finishing uninjured over expanding the performance envelope, then I'm not going to keep any records other than those which my memory may contain.

In all these timed events I have found one truth that applies to me. It was true ten years ago and still true today. It is not about getting a good time. It is about having a good time. That latter is much more important. Why?

It guarantees I will be back for more.

22 – Hobby, Addiction or Obsession?

You now know that I spend one heck of a lot of time on my fitness activities compared to most people. Fourteen years into this I am wondering: Is it a hobby? An addiction? Or an obsession, perhaps? I think that's a sufficiently diverting question for me to pen a short chapter on it. If you disagree feel free to cut straight to the next one and I'll see you there.

I visualise that question as discussing where the needle points to on an imaginary gauge, with the scale marked with Hobby at the left, Addiction in the middle and Obsession on the right. To start with, the needle wasn't anywhere on this scale as fitness for me was none of these; it was an instruction. I had those doctors' words from back in 2006 to think of. One doctor said I wasn't medically fit to fly a plane any longer and the other told me maybe I wouldn't be around in ten years. If that wasn't an instruction to correct the previous fifty years while I still could, then I don't know what it was.

That instruction soon became something of a hobby and started activating that needle. I know exactly when that was: that Magic Moment I described at the end of Chapter 5 when I realised that I was spending time, effort and money on improving my fitness because I wanted to, rather than because I was being told to.

I think over the years since then, the needle on the dial has moved away from the Hobby end and usually points at the Addicted value. I check my weight and bodyfat daily and, as you know, I have limits for both to determine whether or not I'm in my Target Zone. If we are away travelling and I can't do this, I'm always keen to check first morning after we return to see what remedial action is needed to put me back in the zone. If I can't go to the gym for a couple of days, I definitely become a bit grumpy. Holidays excepted of course; but no, actually, delete that, because there aren't many holidays that we've been on in ten or more years where I haven't found a gym in or near where we were staying. I usually check that before booking the place. Yes, that's probably a sign of addiction.

Perhaps having a defined set of numbers for weight and bodyfat places me as being beyond addicted, putting me at the Obsessed end of the scale? I would say no. I know what it is like to be overly fat and the insidious way that bodyfat sneaks up. I never intended to be obese, nor have any of my clients, but the bodyfat goes on when you don't pay attention. Is it therefore beyond an addiction to devote twenty seconds a day to monitor it, to make sure that doesn't happen?

As I mentioned before I like to spend around 30-40 minutes cardio in the morning, 40 minutes on weights in the afternoon or evening and around 15 minutes on abs and stretching most days. That hasn't changed for many years. I took early retirement from full-time employment and set myself up into pretirement as a personal trainer and fitness consultant, and that has seen more and more of my time spent on fitness activities on top of those 90 or so minutes. And if you count my time writing and broadcasting as fitness activities as well, then it's a bigger figure again. This is moving me towards the right on the Addict scale.

This next point probably has Jenny up at the addict level too. There has to be something mighty important happening elsewhere in our lives for us to miss our Saturday morning parkrun. I think the furthest we've travelled to reach a parkrun is three hours' drive or train – six hours travel in total, for a thirty-minute run. And Jenny does that with me to this day despite her being injured and just a spectator. I would point out that I know people who have taken long-haul flights just to do a parkrun (hello David). I think parkrun addiction is a separate condition to fitness addiction.

How do these addictions work together? Which would I do: parkrun or gym, if they were competing activities? The answer without doubt is parkrun. I enjoy them both but of course parkrun can only happen for one half hour per week and I can probably find another time to visit the gym. And parkrun is a Jenny-and-me activity which moves it up the priority list. Does that attitude to parkrun make me less likely to be obsessed with fitness in general and heading to the gym in particular, I wonder?

I feel that having my Target Zone defined and tracking it daily keeps me in the addicted range rather than obsessed, but it could sound a bit obsessive. Why just addicted? Because when my morning weigh in reveals me to be inside my Target Zone, which I try to be for around 75% of the time, then I don't worry about consuming too much of the wrong stuff for that day. I would never turn down a social invitation or the chance for some interesting ale and that applies when I'm in the Target Zone or even just outside, as I know I can return to where I want to within a day or two. That's a situation that I can summarise in another one of my sayings: 'I workout so that I can go out'. That doesn't sound obsessed to me.

If I continually applied restrictions on social gatherings, then I would be worried about myself (as would Jenny) and I wouldn't argue with the obsessive term. It is true that I don't tend to have big pig-out meals anymore and I am a rare visitor to the local chippy, burger shop or kebab van. I would say that is because I am now used to eating more healthily most of the time and do so without thinking; and maybe that is a further sign of fitness addiction.

Once or twice in my fitness life I have noticed that I'm spending rather longer at the gym than I need to as I'm in my Target Zone on weight and fat and there's no particular reason coming up that needs me to be in great shape. I think I'm good at spotting if commitment to fitness and sporting activities are taking over too much of my life, but it creeps up on you – well it does in me, anyway. To ensure it's under control, I've given Jenny a notional electric circuit with a big red warning light connected to a button she can press. The 'Obsession Button' is rarely pressed, but we keep it ready. It doesn't really exist, of course, other than as a concept agreed between us.

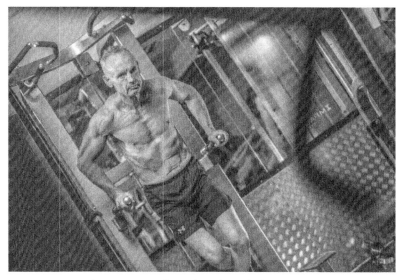

Obsession time? Final workout before contest

However, there are occasions where I've definitely moved the Hobby-Addiction-Obsession needle further to the right. These are specific times, mainly photoshoots or physique contests, when I wanted to be exceptional. These are the times, no more than once or twice a year, when I take my fitness activities to levels beyond that needed purely for health and on to a higher point needed for competitive activity, even if that competition is only with myself. To do this requires effort, dedication and time commitment way beyond the amounts most people would put in. Then is the time to de-wire that Obsession Button.

This is the case with any sport. You have to put the effort and time in and remove or minimise distractions if you're going to achieve success. In those few weeks I am much closer to obsessed than addicted. I won't miss a workout; won't have a cheat meal, or a sneaky beer. I have t-shirt lurking at the back of my wardrobe somewhere that says

'Obsessed is a word used by the lazy to describe the dedicated'. I don't wear it, but I do occasionally think about it in those pre-event weeks.

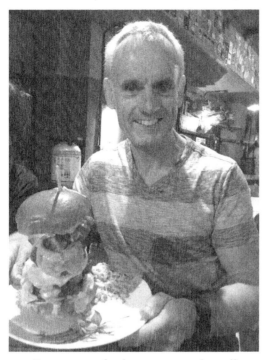

Post-event refeed - not my usual meal!

Once the event is over, I waste no time in returning to my normal state. At that stage I am without doubt substantially within my weight and fat Target Zone with exceptionally low levels of bodyfat compared to my norm.

Without doubt I could have a good couple of weeks on junk food at high quantities before leaving the zone. But I let myself down more sensibly, one or two blow-out meals and back to normal addiction level.

Finally, I think that most of my non-fitness friends would classify me as a fitness addict, especially as they rarely see me in those pre-contest obsessed days. I am sure that many of them realise that lowering the fatness and upping the fitness has quite possibly saved my life, and certainly made it more enjoyable. One or two friends have said that I didn't really need to go all the way to producing the TV shows, popping over to California gyms regularly, attending all the photoshoots and the physique contests, all just in order to get myself fit. Those things are all very well, they say, but are probably neither necessary nor appropriate at my age. Strangely I've heard the same people agree with the sentiment that 'age is just a number', meaning that your age shouldn't be a limiting factor to your activities. I didn't linger on that conflicted viewpoint. I bought them another beer and moved the conversation on.

I reckon the above all proves the needle on the gauge would show that I am addicted to my fitness life and have been so for well over a decade. I agree with that indication. There are many worse things to be addicted to. I can't think of many better.

And I would recommend it to anyone.

23 – The Next Steps

This is the final chapter in Part One and concludes my own story. This is where I should be setting out all my plans and ambitions for the future and the great things I have plans to do to take my fitness ever onward.

But I can't do that as I don't really have any ambitions. That may sound really negative but is not meant to be. I have been so lucky to be able to do everything in fitness that I want to do and many more things that I was able to take advantage of through being in the right place at the right time. I've trained in some of the best gyms in the world, have a cupboard full of trophies from those nine physique contests and made some great friendships along the way. There's nothing left on the fitness aspirational list.

So, without new ambitions, how about simply carrying on as I am? I have no idea how long I can continue with my fitness routine at the current level. I'm 63 now, and I don't have any plan to reduce my commitments to building and maintaining my fitness levels. It will not be lack of a desire that diminishes the effort I put in on my daily workouts. I suspect it will be injuries or other medical setbacks that force it.

The biggest of those medical issues so far is a recent diagnosis of arthritis in both shoulders. The flexibility there is not what it used to be. In particular, the rotational movement is restricted such that I can't press totally vertically any more. On the right side it's about 30 degrees forward of the vertical and about 15 degrees on the left. This condition doesn't affect my daily life, but overhead movements in the gym are restricted and it makes a back squat impossible, a back squat being a leg exercise where a bar is resting across the rear of your shoulders and base of the neck. I can't do that movement any longer because I can't rotate my arms far enough back to hold the bar in place with my hands. Luckily a bar has been invented that helps people with that particular body defect[16], and there are many other exercises that work the same leg muscles.

Was the arthritis caused by my gym training? My consultant couldn't say definitely. Both my mother and grandmother had it, and there are hereditary aspects to the condition. I don't have any siblings to compare with. The advice was given to me relating to gym training was: Continue, 'but don't go too far'. As an aside, I've never considered that to be very useful advice from any medical practitioner on any matter of concern; not until the body is fitted with a strain gauge with a red-shaded zone.

I expect I'll have more medical conditions to contend with later in my sixties and beyond. I'm good at creating alternative exercises and workarounds for mobility problems in my clients and I'm sure that skill is going to be needed for myself as those years pass. And if I can't do everything due to medical issues, let's look at what I can do, and focus on that while trying to rehab the impacted area back up to a better level of function. A saying I use (yes, another one of my sayings) is that: 'if there's something you really want to do, you'll find a way to do it; if there's something you really don't want to do, you'll find an excuse.' I'll find a way to do most of what I want to do.

Since turning sixty, I've noticed that my increases in performance have slowed to a stop for most body parts, and for some have started to slide back. For example, my dumbbell flat bench chest press, which a few years back I was pressing at 36kg, now has a maximum of 30kg. And dumbbell bicep curls have slipped back from 18kg to 16kg. I am talking about ten repetitions here and ensuring good form throughout (there's much more on the detail of these exercises, form and reps in Part Two). I will be continuing my efforts on these exercises as with all others to try to halt and maybe reverse the decline.

The natural loss of muscle as we age is a condition known as sarcopenia – it can be slowed down significantly through good nutrition and exercise but can't be eliminated. Even if I carry on my daily gym visits for another thirty years, my performance will have dropped. I am far fitter at 63 than I was at 33, but don't hand me those 30kg dumbbells for a chest press when I'm 93. Metabolic ageing can be decelerated, but it can't be cancelled.

It's much the same on cardio. I expect to be on the treadmill and cross-trainer in the gym until the day I physically cannot do so, even if the pace eases off. The same is true for parkrun. My fastest parkrun was about 24 minutes, but these days a fast run is about 26.

I don't keep a detailed record but I have already committed to myself to keep below 30 minutes for a 5k for as many years in the future as I can. Running and cycling longer distances are things that I enjoy enormously, but I enjoy them most of all when doing them with Jenny. I probably won't do any more of these events in the future unless Jenny has entered as well. Most of the long runs and bike rides I described in Chapter 21 were with her, and I can't see myself wanting to go solo on these. Jenny and I would definitely would like to run at least one more Marathon du Médoc. It is such a fun event. All we need is a substantial level of recovery from that injury of hers. And we want to do a long cycle ride in the Rockies, one day when her injury recovery permits.

I am still motivated to be the best I can and I'm sure the needle in that Hobby-Addiction-Obsessive gauge is still remaining pointing at Addicted even with that shoulder problem and with the gym and running numbers moving in the wrong direction. I will be entering the physique contest at Muscle Beach soon to give me something to aim for. They don't have an over 63 age group, I'll have to enter the over 45s. I'll be training and competing there with my friend Rob Richley from Southport, and both Jenny and Rob's girlfriend will be flying to LA to watch us. One more contest, Chris? Yes, nine just isn't round enough.

That's enough about me and my own enjoyment from the fitness lifestyle, but how about spreading the word to others? I said at the beginning of Chapter 1 that bringing that message to as many people as I can of my age group is the most important thing I can do to help my age group and society at large. Have I succeeded?

From what I pick up from clients and followers, the answer is yes, so far, and don't stop. I have a string of successful personal training clients from my PT business, so I've certainly passed the message on there. Add to that my TV series, videos, radio, podcasts, members' club and articles and I am doing everything that I can think of to promote increased levels of fitness to those in their second half century.

Perhaps the one idea remaining would be to write a book promoting fitness to my age group. It has taken many more months than I had planned, as I keep getting distracted, but the fact that you are reading it now means that it is complete. And the really important part of the book, where we work on your own fitness, starts over the page.

One of the best ways to a happier, more contented life is to find something you enjoy doing which is good for you. Then, having found it, keep doing it for as long as possible. If you are over fifty, and you know that it would be good for you to increase your fitness levels and decrease your fatness levels, then I'll see you in Part Two.

You've read my journey. Now, let's start on yours!

PART TWO: YOUR STORY

1 – Planning for the Future

Welcome to the second part of this book, and to the journey leading to the next part of your life.

As you no doubt suspect, there's some reading ahead. Can I ask you to make yourself a tea or coffee first? Right now. Any type of tea or regular coffee is fine - instant is perfect, nothing fancy. Make it decaffeinated or herbal tea if this is an evening and you find caffeine disrupts your sleep. If you normally take it with milk or cream, put in half the amount. It's the same with sugar – half the usual amount, please. Don't just skip to the next paragraph, please do this. Right now, as I said. It's an important step which I'll come back to it later.

Great, get comfortable and enjoy the brew while reading. Talking of reading, let me start by discussing the possible reasons why you reading this at all and why you are doing so now at this point in your life. Maybe it's your own realisation that you will be in a better position to enjoy life now and in the decades ahead by changing your fatness or fitness levels now. Perhaps these changes in you are ideas that someone near and dear to you has been suggesting for some time. Another possibility is that, as it was for me, a doctor's warning on your health has brought this issue to the fore. Whatever has prompted you to find yourself here, I am going to make four assumptions, here's the first one: (1) You believe you are overweight and think it would be a good idea to lose some of that weight.

I don't like the word 'overweight'. Your weight at any time is the sum of the weight of your muscles, bodyfat, water in muscles and elsewhere, bones, skin and other organs, and blood and other body liquids. You can't really do much about most of these (no-one has ever asked for their heart or bones to be reduced in mass to reduce their bodyweight) so we'll ignore them for now. On the other hand, you can do a lot about the weight of muscles and intramuscular water, but again you won't want to reduce those in order to save weight. It's the bodyfat that we really want to change to affect our weight, both the fat beneath the skin that makes us bigger and the nastier fat that builds up in the blood vessels and around the internal organs. You were probably thinking just of the first type in that assumption but your heart knows all about the second type and it is likely that if you think you have too much of the first, you probably have too much of the second.

People sometimes ask me for help because they want to help lose fat from a particular location; maybe it's thighs, tummy or upper arms. The answer, which usually disappoints, is that there is no way to 'spot reduce' your bodyfat in this way. As you lose weight the body will choose by itself where to take its fat from and you have as little say in it as you did in telling the body where to store the fat in the first place. In one way it's good that you can't control it; because losing bodyfat as the body determines will include losing a proportion of that nasty internal fat that builds up around the organs, the visceral fat which, as you can't see it, would probably not be on your list of selected fat locations to reduce. But it's massively important for your health that it gets to a lower level.

We'll discuss bodyfat types later, but what I want to do now is restate my first assumption on your views. You know I don't like or use the word 'overweight' very often so I propose a rewording to: (1) You believe your bodyfat levels are too high and think it would be a good idea to lose some of that weight. Agree?

I'll take that as a yes, and I'll venture on to my second assumption: (2) You believe that being fitter would be a good idea too.

Maybe that second assumption hasn't occurred to you so far, and you were just thinking of the first one. If so, I'd like to try to expand your horizon to include the fitness-up element as well as the fatness-down.

Increasing your fitness levels will help you enjoy life, making it possible for you to discover new activities that perhaps you hadn't considered or thought it was too late in your life to attempt. In the longer term, increased fitness will set you up for a mobile and independent life in the years and decades to come. Although fitness and health are not the same thing, you are more likely to have increased health from increased fitness. To confirm that, think if anybody has ever said that they want to get less fit as that will make them healthier?

Look at it this way: the opposite of heading towards increased fitness is to head towards being weak and frail, not an attractive proposition now and worse still thinking of the decades to come. Thanks to a process called sarcopenia, the natural loss of muscle mass as we age, becoming weak and frail happens as the default condition. You can't cancel sarcopenia, but increased fitness levels are a key contributor to delaying it. No one wants to start a bodyfat loss programme hoping to become weaker and less able, giving that unwelcome old sarcopenia a helping hand. If you still think all you want to do is lose bodyfat and you're not so sure about the time and effort needed on the fitness side, then the great news is that an increase in fitness is best achieved in parallel with bodyfat reduction as the tasks involved in pursuing one of those objectives are much the same as those for the other.

Have I convinced you? I hope so. Having those two assumptions nailed, let me add my third assumption – (3) you really want to do something about those first two points and are prepared to put time and effort into making a success of doing so.

I don't care if you've tried before and failed, or if this is your first attempt to improve these aspects of your life. But you have to have a desire to make that change and you acknowledge that the journey will require effort and time on your part. Don't worry about whether you have the amounts of time, effort or willpower to do this; we'll come to that later. You've bought this book, so there's some investment of cash to start off with. What I want from you now is an acknowledgement of that third point: that you know it's going to take some work and commitment on your part.

If you're still on board, that leads to my final assumption on your beliefs – (4) the end result will be worth the effort. I can't guarantee that you'll live a long, happy, mobile and independent life by following my suggestions. But I can say that the chances of that happening are increased with the reduced fatness and fitness levels at levels that your doctor would like to see, rather than being away from those targets. If you don't agree, I'll try the reverse approach again – has anyone ever said that they believe they will live longer through being less fit and more fat?

You're still with me, excellent. We have now rebranded your initial weight-loss idea into a fat-down, fit-up plan. That's the way to think about it from this point onwards. You're not trying to lose weight; you're on a plan to reduce bodyfat and increase body fit. And we know that you are prepared to put time and effort into it as the end result will be worth it. Later on, we'll talk about how not only are the results worth it but the journey can be fun too.

One of the big disadvantages of a book is that it is a one-way flow of information. I can give you concepts, comments, suggestions and even instructions, but I can't get any immediate feedback from you and use that to tailor my next bit of information for you. This makes life difficult for me (don't feel sorry, it's my job) as I can only write for a generic audience.

You know a lot about me, especially if you've read Part One. But what do I know about you? Well, I'm fairly sure that you are over fifty – but you could be any age in that second half-century. Before going on, I want to summarise those assumptions I made about you, and ask you to check that they apply to you.

As a reminder, I'll restate those:

1. You believe your bodyfat levels are too high and think it would be a good idea to lose some of that weight.

2. You believe that being fitter would be a good idea.

3. You really want to do something about those first two points and are prepared to put time and effort into making a success of doing so.

4. You believe the end result will be worth the effort.

Still with me? Excellent, you've acknowledged there is an issue and are keen to work towards resolving it. The rest of this book is designed to help you. Not for you? Maybe have a chat with your GP and see if they agree with your view. But if your GP doesn't agree, then you'll come back here. Agreed?

Most of what I have to say in the remaining chapters are general principles that you can vary depending on your gender, age, height, weight, bodyfat amount and current fitness level. I will try to make my comments as universally applicable as I can, giving guidelines where possible. Please try to remember that I actually don't know you so I can't tailor numbers to meet your exact needs. I'm sure we can work around that together.

But the one set of very important facts about you that we can't work around is that I don't know any physical or medical constraints that you have that would limit your ability to follow my guidance. As a personal trainer I have a duty not to suggest any course of exercise action and dietary adjustment to a client without having medical clearance to do so. That is the first task at the beginning at the personal training relationship when a client discloses all relevant medical data to me, which is when I seek the approval of their GP if needed before going ahead. Such monitoring continues before each session with that client, as I recheck to see if there are any additional medical issues that haven't been mentioned already. We obviously don't have the luxury of doing that in a book, so you're going to have to control this aspect.

Wherever possible I will include alternative forms of exercise that may be able to avoid an issue, perhaps with a different position or emphasis or with alternative equipment. I can supply suggestions and describe the differences but I can't tell you whether they will circumvent any limitation you may have. You're the boss.

In summary, if there's any aspect of what I describe in the chapters that follow that you aren't certain is within your capabilities, then look at any alternatives or discuss it with your GP first. More generally, if you have such concerns or constraints, see your GP first anyway and tell them that you are embarking on a nutrition and exercise plan consisting of cardiovascular and resistance training to both reduce your fatness level (GP will approve) and increase your fitness level (GP will approve again), but you want to check first it is safe for you to do so, and find out if there are any movements you should avoid. You may think this is a waste of your GP's time, since you aren't actually presenting with a current medical problem; but I know they would much rather prevent an issue occurring in you than having to help fix it afterwards.

One thing I won't mention is age limitations. I made a short video[17] for Sun Life called 'Life After Fifty', designed to show that you're never too old to start something new, a saying I firmly believe in. I am far fitter at my current age of 63 than I was at half that number. And my oldest client personal training client (hello again, Mike) is 76 and getting metabolically younger every year. So, there is no blanket exception due to age. Think of the joys of being more mobile and active in five years' time than you are today, then repeat with future periods of five years. But first, as with medical issues and physical limitations, consider your position and review with your GP if you have any doubts. As I said earlier, you're the boss here.

There aren't any gender limitations either. My recommendations work for males and females. The same nutrition approaches encourage bodyfat accumulation, the same activities reduce bodyfat levels and the same exercises improve muscle, whichever gender you are. The numbers will of course be different and I'll discuss that more in the relevant chapters.

A quick point before we go on to your own individual fit-up, fat-down journey. If you've read Part One, you may find some pieces of text in this part seem rather familiar. I've put some of the detail that's common to both parts in the appendices to reduce this. Why the repetition? It's because the recommendations for you are based on my own experiences and research on myself undertaking my own fat-to-fit journey from the age of fifty. One thing you won't find in this Part is any pictures. Part One was about me and stuffed with photos of me. Part Two is about you and I don't have any images of you (yet).

There's nothing in the chapters that follow that I haven't tried and I only recommend actions to you because they were successful when I did them. I believe that the majority of my recommendations will prove similarly successful for the majority of readers. However, I know that everybody is different so I can't guarantee that everything that worked for me in my fat-down, fit-up journey will work for you.

Giving you the knowledge, encouragement and confidence to make a fat-to-fit change as I did is the aim of this part of the book. Let's start with the body part that is most influenced by those three factors and is by far the most important thing you possess in determining the success of your fitness journey.

2 – Starting at the Top

It's important to approach this fat-down, fit-up project with the right mindset. If your brain wants to do something your body will tend to want to follow. That's more notable in the reverse direction. For example, people are more likely to give up while running a race if their head has had enough of it rather than because the legs physically giving up.

The brain and what you think, hope and aspire to, as well as what you dislike and dread, is the most important part of your body in the fitness plan you are now starting. Here are some thoughts that may help in getting (and keeping) your mindset on track.

I would always suggest that the goal of this new project is considered to be a new and upgraded lifestyle, where fitness and fatness levels are now important aspects to you. Adopting this project is the first step in that exciting new lifestyle. It's not a temporary thing. You are making changes now that will create a new way to live the rest of your life. Definitely it's not 'going on a diet'; don't even consider that term because it has such negative and joyless connotations.

It's important to remember that you are doing this lifestyle upgrade for your own benefit. Your body is the most important thing you own, and replacement parts are really hard to obtain at Halfords. You are improving your condition for your life's enjoyment in both the short and long term and you know that the effort involved in doing so is worthwhile. I know you believe this, but if this is sounding a little selfish and self-centred, think how much your loved ones will enjoy and benefit from having you as a fitter person around in the decades ahead than you would otherwise be.

Talking of your nearest and dearest, it's important that those you live with understand why you're doing this, what the expected outcome is and what the journey is likely to involve. For even though it's only you on this project, others will feel the effects – such as the time you are doing more exercise than before, eating differently from how you used to, and thinking in a new and more positive way. A perfectly supporting household will back you through all of this and will not try to encourage you away from your intended track. Not everyone will have such a good setup at home and if that's you, then that makes your task just a little more difficult. I'm not going to become involved in intra-domestic disputes here, but remember to be as kind and understanding of your family and friends as you want them to be to you. In tough times kindness reflects back on itself.

One of the real benefits of face-to-face personal training is accountability. I don't give my clients anything specifically called homework but every week I agree with them what they will be doing to help their fitness project in the 167 hours of the following week that I don't see them. When we meet in that final one hour, we discuss whether those efforts have been successful. That's how it works with personal training but of course, we don't have that accountability system in this book. You are accountable to yourself and should devote time to self-analysis if you are not obtaining the results you expect. I'll offer what guidance I can but you and you alone are responsible for what happens to your body.

One thing I won't be doing in the book is giving you instructions or setting you any rules to follow. I'll give direction, suggestions, advice and perhaps encouragement, but I won't be laying down the law. You're doing this lifestyle upgrade project because you want to and accepting or rejecting any idea from me is your own decision. I believe that the more closely you follow my guidelines the more likely you are to achieve success - and more quickly too; but the adoption of each of my recommendations is totally up to you.

I'm also not going to tell you when to stop. I hope you won't ever want to stop fitness activities entirely because if you do, I've failed in my messaging so far. But there will be a time when you have reached your desired weight, fatness and fitness levels and you move from a 'progress' phase to a 'maintenance' phase. We'll talk more about the approach to this in the last chapter of the book.

You probably want to involve your friends and maybe work colleagues in your plans. This can be a risky area and you need to be careful here. Others may not hold back in perhaps making a joke about your efforts or try to tempt you away from what you want to do. One of my clients told me that his colleagues at work had told him. 'What at your age? You're too far gone for that!' Needless to say, this is the worst kind of feedback from the crew, and you as the captain of your own enterprise need to divert all power to the shields to deflect any harm to your good intentions. I do not of course know what your friends and work colleagues are like but be aware of that unwelcome possibility. If you get any negativism from those quarters be nice to them. They don't have your interests at heart and are nowhere near as important to your long-term future as you are.

I'm not going to ask you to follow 100% of my suggestions for 100% of the time. That just isn't going to work. You'll make a success of it by following most of my recommendations, most of the time. The higher the percentages are, the sooner the desired outcome is likely to be achieved. But high levels of adherence are not possible in the real world. You have a life outside the lifestyle upgrade programme. Live your real life but always keep an eye on the fitness aspects of what you are doing. Initially you will have to remember to do that but soon it will become second nature. I don't know you or your situation well enough to be any more specific at the outset but I'll have suggestions later on.

From time to time, you will have days that really are in contravention to the spirit of the project – I know I do. This is similar to what I discussed in the last paragraph, but more so. These are days when far too much of the bad stuff is consumed and far too little of the good stuff is being done. That's fine – I expect such days in your plan... (Delete that; you are in charge.) That's fine; you expect such days in your plan and you will pick yourself up, brush yourself off, and start all over again. You'll be back on the fitness wagon the next day, provided you acknowledge that the falling off happens, was for an enjoyable purpose, but is temporary. It's amazing how quickly a really bad day gets forgiven by the body when your norm is good days.

Be realistic about progress. Those extra pounds didn't go on overnight and they aren't going to come off immediately. But the good news is that you can remove decades' worth excess bodyfat in much less time than it took to acquire. I was putting on bodyfat for three decades but lost that excess in three years; and the scales showed me making real progress within the first week, progress that continued for the three years.

The likelihood of success of any person's fat-down and fit-up project can be viewed in terms of their ability to prioritise long-term satisfaction over short-term satisfaction most of the time. You want to be fit, to be at a recommended weight and to be healthy for the coming decades more than you want that jam doughnut now. Most of the time.

A final point on mindset, and like everything else I have mentioned, it comes directly from my own experience. One day, due to a business trip, I couldn't find the time to do the exercise that I had planned for that day. I was stunned to realise I was regretting not being able to do so. In that one second I discovered that I was by that stage doing all the fitness stuff because I wanted to, not because I had to. I call it my Magic Moment; it crept up on me unnoticed about two months after starting. From that point on, it was never a chore to undertake my exercise or eat nutritiously. Guess what? I predict you will have a Magic Moment too. It will stun you too. I can't say when the moment will occur. Maybe it will be at a similar point in time to mine – just a couple of months after you started your own fitness project; which you have of course already started.

Really? Yes, you have already started. That cup that previously held a warm beverage with only 50% of your previous level of milk, cream and sugar was your first step. It would be good if you could take all your tea and coffee like that from now on and move to none of those additions when you can.

Doing that would probably be an upgrade in the quality of your beverage. The next chapter is devoted to expanding on that topic, improving more of your nutrition, by giving you the information you need to make healthier choices on food and drink.

It's a big subject and a big chapter. Get comfortable; maybe with a second cuppa? Perhaps a decaff, if the last one was a strong coffee?

3 – Basic Nutrition

The choices people make on the types and quantities of food and drink consumed are of vital importance to them living healthy lives. Yet many people know relatively little about this area, a fact which occurs to me most often when I meet a new personal training client and discuss this subject. It is really more of a society issue than a fault with an individual client; it stuns me how little is taught about even basic healthy eating concepts in schools. And how many messages will you see on an average evening in front of the TV promoting healthy eating ideas and how many promoting less nutritious food to buy?

You're not here to receive a presentation on society and healthy nutrition from me. You are here to follow my plan to increase your fitness levels and reduce your fatness levels. However, in order to do that, I am going to give you some basic nutrition concepts that most people don't know but really should.

Over 50% of your success on the plan will be due to the good choices you make on food and drink. I was obese by the age of fifty thanks in part to my decades of poor nutrition choices. I reversed that high level of bodyfat in me in a couple of years by changing the food and drink I chose, as well as increasing exercise.

This information isn't designed to go into any more detail than is needed to help you succeed on the plan, with maybe an interesting or personal observation or two on the way. It absolutely isn't a detailed study of nutrition; if it was, the book would be ten times as thick.

I am going to use a nutrition panel from a packaged food item as my guide to make this description as practical as possible. You may find it helps your understanding to have some packaged foods to hand as we go through this. It can be anything with a nutrition label. I have a pack of oats to look at in front of me.

Each packaged food item has to have a nutrition label, and the type of information provided on it is governed by law. All this is designed to help people make better food choices.

There may well be two columns of numbers on any nutrition panel, one for a standardised amount (say per 100g), to help comparison with other products and one for a typical serving as judged by the manufacturer (perhaps per 40g). Manufacturers sometimes use a small serving as being typical so watch out for this; the pack of oats I am looking at suggests 40g is typical, which is actually under two-thirds of what I normally prepare for myself every morning.

Calories

The energy value of food and drink is measured in calories. The more calories your food and drink supply, the more energy it gives you; and the energy you burn up in everything you do is also measured in calories.

The comparison between the in and the out is often called the Energy Equation, the balance of which results in bodyweight up if you are net storing calories, or bodyweight down if you are net burning calories. Your surplus of bodyfat today is probably the accumulated energy you have consumed and not used over the past years or decades.

The first number shown in the nutrition panel is for the energy content of the food, which you know as calories but correctly called kilocalories, so you will see the abbreviation 'kcal'. There's an alternative measuring system used in several countries called kilojoules, abbreviated as 'kJ'. You can ignore the kJ information (unless of course you are in one of those countries, in which case everything I say about calories in this book needs to be increased upwards by multiplying by 4.2).

All food is made up of water, micronutrients and macronutrients. Let's look at each.

Water

I'll talk about the water in food first, as that is dealt with quickly here.

I find it interesting that even the driest-looking food items usually contain some water. You can see this for yourself from a nutrition panel by adding together the grams shown for the different nutrients and comparing the totals with the 'per' figure at the top. It probably will fall short and that gap is water. For example, on the pack of oats I have to hand, the total of the nutrients listed below the calorie number comes to 88g per 100g – meaning that the missing 12g is water.

I have more to say about the water you drink over the course of the day, but that's coming later.

Micronutrients

This topic is also easily discussed so I'll tackle them next. Micronutrients are substances needed in tiny amounts by the body, specifically vitamins, minerals and other chemicals that occur naturally in a food. Tiny amounts, that is, compared to the macronutrients coming next.

You probably know that an orange is known for its high level of Vitamin C. There's a whole load more good stuff in an orange of course such as some Vitamin A and useful minerals including calcium and potassium and antioxidants. Those are all examples of micronutrients in food.

Every micronutrient has a daily target amount to be consumed, known as its Nutrient Reference Value, or NRV. You may see this on nutrition panels including the amount of the nutrient supplied by the food and the percentage it meets of the NRV. It's outside the scope of this book to go into more detail on this.

There is a micronutrient gap in many people's diets. That's a term used to describe the difference between the level of micronutrients recommended and the level consumed. In my case I try to rely on my varied diet to meet most of my micronutrient needs. To be sure that I have reduced the chances of falling down the gap I take a good combined multivitamin and multimineral tablet once per day, as I don't want to fall short on some of these minute but vital goodies. If you believe you would be missing out in the same way, try the same approach as me.

Macronutrients

This is next and it is the fun bit.

There are three main macronutrients: protein, carbs (which is easier to say than 'carbohydrates' and much easier to type from now on) and fats. These nutrients together are called 'macro' as they occur in comparatively large quantities in a typical diet, macro being the opposite of micro. These are particularly important to you as the source of calories in all food is from its macronutrients.

You can see there is a separate gram figure for each of the three macronutrients on your nutrition panel. My oats contain 11g of protein, 60g of carbs and 8g of fats per 100g of oats.

You may also notice that sugars, a type of carb, and saturated fat, a type of fat, have a separate listing on your nutrition panel. The grams for these two form parts of the bigger numbers. With my oats, it is carbs 60g of which sugars are 1g, and fats 8g of which saturates are 2g. Look at the nutrition panels of the foods you have to check you can find this information.

Macronutrient: Protein

I'll start with protein first as it's the easiest to discuss. Protein is of primary importance in helping the body rebuild itself. In fact, 'primary importance' is the translation of the Greek word from which we derive the word protein.

The functions of protein in the body are all the building, repair and support functions. In particular, for muscle, bones, tissues and cells, together with hormone creation, supporting the immune system, promoting a healthy metabolism, stabilising blood sugars and assisting the recovery from sport or illness. As you can see protein is a vital nutrient for the growth and continuing health of the body. Protein also helps you to feel fuller and curbs appetite, two effects of great help to those trying to eat less and eat better.

 It is also a nutrient that isn't stored in the body. Protein should be included in everyone's daily diet whether they trying to lose weight or not.

Top sources of protein are eggs, meat, fish and dairy products. Egg white is a particularly good source of protein and indeed the German word for protein translates to 'egg white' in English. It is often hard to obtain sufficient protein in the diet and low-carb protein shakes can help. When mixed with water they can add substantial numbers of protein grams without fat and sugars.

Vegan sources of protein include most beans, seeds, lentils, quinoa and nuts. It is harder for the vegan to find protein sources but it can be done.

Macronutrient: Fats

We are talking about fat here as the macronutrient found in food, sometimes called dietary fat to save any confusion with the fat on and inside the body, which can be called bodyfat.

Fats come in various types. I'll start with the worst to get it out of the way quickly, then work upwards in goodness.

Trans Fats

The worst type of fats is trans fats. Your body's insides do not like these. Keep an eye out for them on nutrition labels and ingredients lists of processed foods, where the word to look for (and avoid) is 'hydrogenated', as well as the term trans fats itself. Most food manufacturers are reducing or eliminating them but sadly they are still allowed in the UK, unlike some European countries and US states which have banned them.

There is no recommended level of these in your diet, just zero. If you see it on a label or on an ingredients list, run a mile; not literally, but do put it down and take something else instead.

Saturated Fats

These are a type of fats that most nutritionists, although not all, say are bad for you. The UK Government believes them to be notably bad amongst fats, which is why there is a dedicated 'of which' number for saturated fats on the nutrition panel.

Most experts believe that saturated fat raises the level of LDL cholesterol in the bloodstream. LDL is the 'bad' cholesterol, a term you may have heard. Too much of that builds plaque up which restricts the flow in the arteries and many believe there is a link from that to an increased risk of heart disease.

Foods that are high in saturates include fatty cuts of meat, chicken skin, whole-fat dairy, coconut and palm oils, processed meats, fried food, chocolates, ice cream, cakes, and pies and pastries of all types.

Unsaturated Fats

Most people agree that there are good types of fats and they are called unsaturated. These are found in oily fish (tuna, mackerel, salmon, trout, sardines) as well as good quality oils, nuts and avocados.

Two reasons why I'm not a massive fan of these: firstly, not all unsaturated fats are seen by everybody as healthy. For example, seeds used as the basis for vegetable oils may start out healthy but the processing of them to produce the oil results in a product that can cause inflammation in the body.

Secondly, beyond dispute, all fats are very calorie dense. Each gram of fat in a food contains more than double the calories of a gram of protein or carbs, and that includes the good fats. That is a lot of energy to consume if you're on an unlimited unsaturated fat regime.

Assuming there are none of those nasty trans fats around, the unsaturated ones make up the remainder of the fats on the label. Reminding you of my oats nutrition panel: 'fats 8g of which saturates are 2g' means that unsaturated fats are the other 6g.

Macronutrient: Carbs

Carbs are vital for the body providing energy for the brain and other organs to function. Just as with saturated fats, you will see that the sugars number is listed separately on nutrition labels from the other carbs.

I'll talk about the sugars first, and why this is such a focus in bodyfat reduction.

Sugars

When the weight loss industry started around the 1950s, fat was seen as the bad-guy nutrient. You were being advised to drastically reduce your fat intake with no advice on limiting sugar. Wind the clock forward fifty years or so, and the situation isn't far from reversed. There are many diets today recommending you to severely lower sugar levels while proposing no limits on the fat intake.

Which is the real bad guy? Actually, they both are. I advise you to limit both fats and sugars, although I'm not recommending an extreme reduction in either to the levels proposed by advocates of views that 'fat is the real demon' or 'sugar is the real demon'.

What is bad about sugar? Sugar is of use in providing short-term energy because it enters the bloodstream very soon after eating; it is a 'fast carb'. The speed of transition from being eaten to appearing in the bloodstream is why long-distance cyclists and marathon runners consume concentrated sugar gels to produce short-term energy that is used by the body very rapidly as fuel.

But if that energy from the sugar isn't used for fuelling your activity very quickly or there is too much sugar, the body can't cope with it. It will then promote the growth of bodyfat and can lead to diabetes and other nasty outcomes. We don't need to eliminate sugars totally from the diet but instead we may want to limit the amount. It is to help with this that sugars are listed separately from other carbs on food nutrition panels.

Sugars are found in many foods including liquids. Sugars can both be naturally occurring (such as in fruit or honey) or added in manufacture, such as in sweets and chocolates, biscuits and cakes, ice creams, sodas and jam.

Sugar comes in a variety of names on ingredients lists. These include caramel, honey, anything followed by syrup; and if it ends in -ose, its likely to be a sugar. Don't be tricked into thinking natural-sounding sugars like honey, agave syrup and maple syrup are better. The body doesn't recognise the difference between them and refined sugars, so they all break down and function in the same way.

The worst foods are those that are high in both fats and in sugars. You can probably work out that I'm looking at you, jammy creamy sugared doughnuts, and anything from nearby in the supermarket such as chocolates, cakes, pastries and ice cream. Yes, all the sweet and lovely stuff.

Non-sugar carbs

I'm not going to say too much about non-sugar carbs, but you may be interested in the fact that all carbs get converted into sugar by the body eventually, and the sugar ends up affecting your blood. Maybe you've heard of blood sugars and that's where that term comes from. The slower that conversion process is the better for the body, as it really doesn't like dealing with fast-converting carbs as I mentioned earlier. Sugar itself is the fastest (therefore potentially the naughtiest) carb, of course. That's why I picked on him in particular, earlier.

The slower non-sugar carbs are found in many foods including vegetables, bread, pasta, cereals and rice. There are various speeds of breakdown, and as a guideline the more natural a product is, the slower and therefore better it is. For example, wholemeal bread is a slower carb than white bread.

There is a table called the glycaemic index, which shows all different carbs in descending order of speed of conversion. These are easily found online, and I recommend you take a look.

To make life a little easier nutrition panels don't divide non-sugar carbs into various speeds of conversion. A carb is either a sugar or it's not. That's it.

Other Nutrition Facts

I've talked about a few things that are very important to your fatness-down, fitness-up project – calories, protein, fats (including saturates) and carbs (including sugars). And by now you know where to find all this information on a nutrition label. Is there anything else of interest on the nutrition side to be aware of?

Plenty; but these aren't so vital to know about as the points already covered. They are of interest and I would like you to be mindful of them in your selection of your food and drink items.

Fibre

Fibre is sometimes given on labels and sometimes not. It's another 'grams per' item, just like protein, fats and sugars, and some people call it a macronutrient. The reason I don't worry too much about fibre is that it passes through the body mainly undigested, and the energy content does not get absorbed by the body, so it has no effect on blood sugar. I ignore the calories that come from fibre for this reason.

So, is fibre worth having? Absolutely; fibre keeps the digestive system working well and helps ensure your toilet visits are, ahem, nice and regular. Fibre from vegetables also helps to maintain an abundance and diversity of the good bacteria in our gut, which are important for overall health, and indeed it may also help with weight loss.

Fibre adds bulk to food contributing to your feeling full and so lowering the temptation to eat more. You find fibre particularly in good cereals, fruit and vegetables, and grains. There's 9g per 100g in my oats, for example.

Salt

Salt is something worth keeping low in your diet. Most foods contain salt, even if you don't think they do, and it is always listed on nutrition labels. Salt of course makes you thirsty (that's why salted peanuts and crisps are offered in pubs), but the worst effect is on blood pressure. Increased consumption of salt leads to high blood pressure, which isn't good for the heart.

I keep my salt down by the simple approach of never actually adding salt to anything – but I don't worry about the salt that occurs within a food item.

Artificial Sweeteners

These aren't exactly health foods, and I choose to limit them whenever I can. Saccharin had been found to be a possible cause of cancer in some animals but not in humans. Other common ones are aspartame, acesulfame-K and sucralose. These have been given clean bills of health by authorities around the world but concerns remain. In particular research has shown that they can disrupt gut bacteria and therefore hamper weight loss.

Most food experts are however happier about stevia which, like everything else I've mentioned in this paragraph, contains no calories, and is an entirely natural ingredient. Do your research if you're concerned about artificial sweeteners.

Sugar Alcohols

Also called polyols, these are a sweetener substitute for sugar.

Most are natural, such as xylitol. Really, it's natural – but have you ever seen such a name that sounds like it's made in a laboratory? Sugar alcohols, including xylitol, are partially resistant to digestion, give little energy to the body and have negligible effects on blood sugar. Since they are very sweet, they are usually found in tiny quantities, and that small amount can be a good substitute for sugar.

Most authorities say they aren't harmful despite containing the two words 'sugar' and 'alcohol'. If it ends in -ol, it's probably a sugar alcohol. Unless it's ethanol which is another word for…

Alcohol

This is something I urge you to limit while on the plan. A pint of beer has 200 calories, and a wine bar glass of wine anything from 175 to 350. Since there are significant calories in it some people consider alcohol a macronutrient.

The calories in alcohol are often called 'empty calories' as they contain nothing of nutritional value. There's no fat, virtually zero protein, and often not much actual sugar in drinks. The sweeter it is, the more likely it is to contain extra sugar. Sweet wine has more sugar than dry, red wine, for example.

Tea and Coffee

Tea and coffee have no calories and can have health benefits. Green tea is known for many micronutrients, some due to its lack of processing. Herbal teas aren't actually teas, but leaves from herb plants. And again, there are micronutrients to be had and no calories too.

Coffee is of course particularly high in caffeine, which is a stimulant and actually helps the body utilise energy that is stored in fat cells. It causes the heart rate to rise and can leave you too alert to sleep if taken in the evening.

Adding milk, cream and/or sugar brings calories along, so it's far better to learn to have these beverages without.

Milk

Milk from cows contains calories, including protein, fats – including saturated – and sugar. It's rich in micronutrients. Indeed, it contains everything needed by youngsters starting out in life. Young cows, that is.

Skimmed milk has less fat, but more of the non-fat milk to make up the volume – and it is that non-fat milk where the sugar lives. The sugar in milk is called lactose and the majority of people, about 70%, including me, have some level of intolerance to its effects. I minimise the amount of milk I consume for that reason. You can Google the effects of lactose intolerance if you are interested.

Goat milk is an alternative that some people prefer. It has a different range of micronutrients to cows', but the big change is lower levels of lactose (still the same amount of sugar, just lower in lactose).

By the way, items like almond milk, coconut milk and other milk from seeds and nuts aren't really milk. You cannot sit on a stool and milk a coconut. It is actually the nut itself, ground up and mixed with water.

Fruit

Fruit is particularly interesting as most fruits contain high levels of fructose, fruit sugar, which is one of the types of sugar that are most likely to be unhealthful.

But fruits also contain lots of natural minerals, vitamins, fibre and natural chemicals that are good for the body. The skins of fruits contain less sugar and are usually the healthiest part. That's one reason why a pear is a better choice for you than the same weight of pineapple. You don't eat the low-sugar part (the skin) of the pineapple - you don't, do you?

Berries are particularly good. They are excellent providers of antioxidants, and of course, relative to their size, there's loads of skin on them (think of the shape of a raspberry or blackberry).

Non-packaged items

One aspect I haven't talked about is that wide range of foods available that don't bear a nutrition panel. These are single ingredient foods, and usually much healthier than their more processed, multi-ingredient counterparts. Examples of single-ingredient foods are fruit and veg, meat, fish and eggs. You won't see a label on an orange: 'Ingredients – umm, an orange'. So how do you derive the nutrition information for that? What are the calories, protein, sugars and fats on these non-packaged items?

Well, you now know that the fact that they are sold as single food items rather than processed indicates they are more likely to be healthy, but it's no guarantee. For example, there can be a lot of fat on some cuts of meat and you may need to limit fruits due to the high sugar content. You can use MyFitnessPal, my favourite app for this kind of information; or just Google 'nutrition in an orange'.

Juicing

This is something that is a personal issue of mine. Yes, it's okay to juice your vegetables; but you would be missing out on some of the fibre and a lot of micronutrients that live in the bits you are discarding. I would rather you ate a real broccoli then the liquid extracted from one.

My real concern is with fruit juice. This often contains all the bad stuff and precious little of the good stuff from the fruit. This applies if you juice at home, just as if you had purchased a carton. An orange is good for you. It has sugar but there's fibre and lots of vitamins, minerals and antioxidants. If you juice it, you lose much of the good parts but preserve all the sugar. And think of quantity; you would only eat one orange but you would juice maybe six to get a decent amount to drink. That's all the sugar from six oranges. It makes me shudder to think about it; and you too, I hope.

Check out the nutrition label on a carton of orange juice next time you're in a supermarket. See if there are any grams of anything except sugar; then put it back on the shelf.

To end this chapter, a few final tips on nutrition and eating generally:

1. If you're going to eat something that isn't that healthy, try to limit the amount. Fancy a big bar of chocolate? Yes. Fancy eating two? Maybe. How about ten, right now? No. The pleasure drops off with quantity. But there are the same calories, fat and sugar in the (unpleasant) tenth bar as there was in the (lovely) first.

    The same applies to anything – take wine. You don't want to drink ten glasses do you? You may be too pickled to give a sensible comment by that stage, but the answer is no. As the pleasure decreases the calories continue straight upwards.

    I call this my DROP law – the Diminishing Returns Of Pleasure. Consume one of the naughty items, then DROP the rest.

2. If you are going to eat or drink something that isn't that healthy for you, select a high-quality product. Make it worth the calories, the sugar, the fat – or whatever.

    Try some craft hand-made beer from a local brewer rather than rubbish lager created by the tanker-full in a factory. Try artisanal bread from the local baker instead of a supermarket pack of white sliced. Savour the quality by eating it slowly. I call this the QNQ rule – Quality, Not Quantity.

3. The food traffic light system on packets is a great help in planning your eating. It isn't perfect since it measures by weight, which includes water. For example, an item could be labelled as low-sugar when in fact sugar represents most of the calories because much of the weight is water.

    However, the four aspects shown in colour are all important to minimise in your die: overall fats, saturated fats, sugar and salt. I suggest you select products with green as much as possible and allow an amber or two as well. An approach I take is: 'If you see any red, take something instead'.

    Bear in mind that the level of the red may well be less when combined with other food items to form the meal. For example, mixed nuts have a high percentage of calories from fats and so they are marked red. However, I usually mix those in a meal with high-carb oats and berries and high-protein shake (all of which are low in fats). Adding the ingredients together removes the red warning. If all the ingredients from the meal were in one packet, there would be no red.

4. Try to make eating a notable event in your daily life and put the times for it in your daily to-do list if you have one. And have a go at resisting the temptation to eat while you are moving (walking, driving or on public transport – I'll let you off flying) or doing something else (reading, internet, TV).

   All those are distractions which lead you to both (1) not really enjoying the pleasure of your food, and (2) eating more than you really intended. It is perhaps an overused word, but I can summarise my point here by advising to eat mindfully; which is, of course, the opposite of mindlessly.

As I said at the start, this chapter isn't intended to give you all possible information relating to nutrition. However, understanding these messages and using them to help in your choices of food and drink will help you succeed in the plan. I've put some simple categories of food choice as good, ok, not good in Appendix C.

Let's turn to the plan itself next.

4 – Introduction to the Plan

I call my fit-up and fat-down lifestyle upgrade plan the 'Fat to Fit at Fifty' plan. I like alliteration and the name describes exactly what it does, so I've also used it for the title of the book.

I have arranged the plan into three stages. You start at Stage One, and then (if you need to) move to Stage Two and then ease off in Stage Three. Stage One has all the elements needed to enable success on your fat-down, fit-up plan. You can be 100% successful on your fat-down and fit-up plan by staying in Stage One. In this stage you don't need to keep daily notes or perform any calculations. There is no calorie counting and no measuring of food or exercise. Stage One trusts you to be good.

You may notice that this goes against some of my principles relating to success, where I have said that you are more likely to achieve success with numbers written down and progress noted over time. So, there is some data, just two numbers you do have to note, and only once a week. That's all you need at Stage One to monitor your progress.

Stage One advises you to be good and tells you how to do so. The activities for you to do are much the same in Stage One and Stage Two, but in Stage One I'm not asking you to keep records. Stage Two has more for you to do in terms of counting nutrition numbers, noting activity and updating spreadsheets. If you don't like the sound of that, then make Stage One successful for you and you never move to Stage Two.

In Stage One is that I am trusting you to do the good things that I describe. That's the fundamental principle. If you can get to your goals without taking on the admin of Stage Two that is brilliant. It really is. I'll be very happy if you never need Stage Two. In that case there will be many chapters that follow that you don't need to read, and that's fine.

I suggest you to try Stage One for a period of two weeks. If after that time you're not making steady progress towards your targets, then I need to be a little stricter with you and off you go to Stage Two. However, if you succeed in making progress towards your targets in those initial two weeks you will be in a great place to continue to follow Stage One guidelines and Stage Two can stay ignored.

As I've said you know you're making progress on Stage One if you are heading towards your goals. You will only know if you are doing that if you have goals and the best goals are the ones you set yourself. And to determine your goals I suggest you need one item of equipment, body composition monitor scales.

This is an upgrade to the traditional bathroom scales. The technology involved in these scales is called bioelectrical impedance. A tiny electric voltage is sent through you and the timing of it passing through your body tissues is measured. As well as weight, a body composition monitor will give you additional data: muscle mass, bone mass, percentage water, visceral fat level, metabolic age are all typical variables shown, and I have no problem with you monitoring all of these. But to keep the admin burden down, I'm interested in two things only: your overall weight and bodyfat percentage. Make sure your new scales support at least those two variables. The scales I use are from Tanita, but other suppliers are of course available. Some of the newer models include ones include Bluetooth connectivity that can synchronise data with Excel.

Once you have the scales, you are ready to set some targets.

5 – Setting Your Targets

How are you going to measure success on your journey? There are many possible ways, both objective and subjective.

The subjective ones would include: I look better in the mirror, my partner says I'm looking fitter, I don't tire as easily, my sleep is improved. I am sure there are a few more you could add relevant to your own situation.

Those are all good feelings and the aims of your lifestyle upgrade include being able to say all those things. I prefer an objective approach with numbers, because if you can measure it you can improve it. That's something I say (and do so annoyingly frequently).

So, what can we measure? Again, there are several things: time to walk or run a set distance, weight you can lift, how long can you jog until you heart rate reaches a certain number, how many push-ups can you do, are some examples. You can probably think of more and, once again, these measures should all improve over the coming weeks and months.

You said you wanted to reduce your bodyfat. Well, you didn't say that exactly, but I suggested it at the very beginning and you carried on reading, which I take as acceptance. We covered this in Chapter 1, but to recap: as someone's overall weight comes down, the situation that usually applies is the weight will be lost across muscle and fat at an approximately equal rate (lose x% of your bodyfat amount, you will lose x% of your muscle amount). That's not what you want. You don't want to end up with low levels of bodyfat, but unfit, scrawny and frail because of low levels of muscle. We want to monitor that, as your overall weight goes down, you lose a higher percentage of bodyfat than muscle. Indeed, you don't want to lose muscle at all and gaining a little would be much better.

That leads to the two key things I recommend that you measure: overall weight and bodyfat percentage. Assuming both of these are currently higher than you would like, then the aim is to bring them both down. I'm going to ask you to write down four numbers plus a couple of dates: your current values for these two measurements, and your planned target values.

Let's set some initial values for your own Fat to Fit at Fifty project.

Use your new body composition analysis scales here and make sure you are familiar with the way the scales operate, specifically in terms of displaying overall weight and bodyfat percentage. You should input your basic data: age, height, gender and (if it asks) you are not an athlete (sorry). Always use the same scales on the same bit of hard floor (not carpet) and take your readings at the same time of day, wearing nothing. If you plan to do this first thing in the morning, which is the best and also the most convenient time for many, then wait until then to continue this chapter. Sleep well.

Good morning! Scales time and grab a pen too. If you are accustomed to using stones and pounds, and can't bear to move away from that, then that's fine, we can live with that. But if you can be persuaded to convert to pounds on their own, or kilograms, then can I suggest you make that change now? It may be much easier later on.

Start by writing in the current values for these:

STARTING WEIGHT:		STARTING BODYFAT %:		STARTING DATE:	

Now we need to set some targets. Rather than take these from a wish list or just a guess, let's put some reasonableness in here.

The choice of your target values on weight, bodyfat percentage and date is up to you. If you select the target it becomes your choice and you 'own' that target. You are more likely to succeed by choosing a target number yourself rather than having one imposed on you.

Firstly, overall weight. To start off, here are the UK Department of Health and Social Care guidelines on healthy weight. For these guidelines, I show the minimum and maximum values of the ranges of healthy weight. It's the same numbers for healthy weight ranges by height irrespective of gender.

Height (ft-in)	Height (cm)	Target Weight – st:lb	Target Weight lb	Target Weight kg
4-11	150	6:08 – 8:12	92 – 124	41.6 – 56.3
5-0	152	6:10 – 9:01	94 – 127	42.7 – 57.8
5-1	155	7:00 – 9:06	98 – 132	44.4 – 60.1
5-2	157	7:03 – 9:10	101 – 136	45.6 – 61.6
5-3	160	7:06 – 10:01	104 – 141	47.4 – 64.0
5-4	163	7:10 – 10:06	108 – 146	49.2 – 66.4
5-5	165	7:13 – 10:10	111 – 150	50.4 – 68.1
5-6	168	8:03 – 11.02	115 – 156	52.2 – 70.6
5-7	170	8:06 – 11:05	118 – 159	53.5 – 72.2
5-8	173	8:10 – 11:11	122 – 165	55.4 – 74.8
5-9	175	8:13 – 12:01	125 – 169	56.7 – 76.6
5-10	178	9:03 – 12:07	129 – 175	58.6 – 79.2
5-11	180	9:06 – 12:11	132 – 179	59.9 – 81.0
6-0	183	9:11 – 13.03	137 – 185	62.0 – 83.7
6-1	185	10:00 – 13.07	140 – 189	63.3 – 85.6
6-2	188	10:04 – 13.13	144 – 195	65.4 – 88.4
6-3	191	10:09 – 14:05	149 – 201	67.5 – 91.2
6-4	193	10:12 – 14:09	152 – 205	68.9 – 93.1

I suggest taking the top-end value from the healthy range if your current weight is significantly above that top end of the healthy weight range. So, if you are age 55, 5 feet 7 inches tall, weigh 80kg, and have a bodyfat percentage of 30%, I suggest you take 72kg as your weight target (rounded down from 72.2). When you reach that target and if you feel you are happy to head further downwards, then consider doing so and select a new target at that time.

Secondly, bodyfat percentage. There are several different sources for reference data on this, but the numbers don't vary by more than 1% across those sources. Here's an average of them showing healthy ranges of bodyfat by percentage of overall weight:

Age	Female	Male
40-59	23% – 33%	11% – 21%
60-79	24% – 35%	13% - 24%

I suggest taking the top-end value from the healthy range if your bodyfat percentage is significantly above that top end of the healthy percentage range. So, if you are a 55-year-old male with a bodyfat percentage of 30%, I suggest you take 21% as your target. Just as with the weight, when you reach that target and if you feel you are happy to head further downwards, then consider doing so and select a new target at that time.

If you aren't significantly over the top end of the range numbers for weight and/or bodyfat today, then maybe start with a lower-number target; but it's your choice and you should feel free to choose different targets from within the healthy range if you prefer.

A note on these target ranges: it's best to check with your GP what the healthy range is that applies to you if you have any specific medical or physical conditions that make you think that the numbers in the target tables may not be appropriate for you. Show your GP this section of the book if that helps.

Finally, you should work out a realistic date when you can reach your targets. I have found that 1 lb (0.5 kg) per week works well for most people; it did for me, and does so for my personal training clients. It is a sustainable rate that results in a notable rate of reduction while being manageable in the real world.

Some people think that is a low rate and it doesn't sound very much at first reading. My view is that it's much better to choose a 1 lb a week weight loss that you sustain for a year rather than an overly optimistic 2 lb a week loss that leaves you miserable after a month and you give up on the plan. By the way, 1 lb a week isn't slow. That is 52lb or 26kg a year of course and that's not a small number. Weight loss is rarely a straight line but it's easiest to assume at this stage that it could be in order to establish a target date.

Going to back to our previous example, our 80kg person has selected 72kg as a target; that's 8kg of loss. At a rate of 0.5kg/week that gives 16 weeks from now as the target date.

So, combining the rate of 0.5 kg /1 lb per week with your starting and target weight, you will be able to calculate a target date. If it needs rounding make it a whole number of week because decimals of weeks are just too painful to work with!

You should now be able to grab that pen and put numbers in these three boxes:

TARGET
WEIGHT:

TARGET
BODYFAT %:

TARGET
DATE:

Well done. Do you feel you can 'own' these numbers and can work towards achieving them with me? If not, revise them. It's important you feel the numbers are your own choice and realistic for you.

One piece of terminology I am going to use is to define two separate body states you could be in and you should understand that you will always be in one or the other. I describe those states as being inside Target Zone or outside it. Inside your Target Zone is defined as being at or lower than both the numbers shown above in the target boxes for weight and bodyfat percentage. If you are higher than one or both of those then you are outside your Target Zone. Obviously, you are just starting on this plan, so you will be outside the zone now.

How are you going to travel from being at the starting numbers to that target set? A question that can now be restated as 'How do you get into the Target Zone?'

Moving from outside the Target Zone to inside it is what the Fat to Fit at Fifty plan is all about. Time to look at the guidelines I want you to apply in Stage One.

6 – Stage One: The Twelve Guidelines

There are twelve guidelines I want you to follow for Stage One. Twelve guidelines do not sound like very many to change your life forever. But they can, and the closer you adhere to them the quicker that change will be.

1. 12-hours on, 12-hours off

   Plan your days such that you have a 12-hour overnight period when you don't consume anything with calories. So that means water, black, green and herbal tea and coffee are fine. Obviously, that is sleep time plus some added awake time at either end. 8pm to 8am is an example of a nothing-consumed 12-hour period. It doesn't have to be the same twelve hours each day so you need to plan when you should schedule this. For example, if you know you must have breakfast at 7am tomorrow, then plan for your last meal to be at 7pm tonight.

2. Eat less

   In the twelve hours that you are eating and drinking, try to consume less food and drink overall. Eat smaller portions than you are used to and eat more slowly. You only feel full 20 minutes after you have eaten enough to make you feel full, so don't eat until you feel full. Try noting if you feel full 20 minutes after a smaller-than-usual meal and you may be surprised.

3. Keep the good stuff up

    While consuming less food overall, keep the protein and fibre
    up (chicken, lean meat, fish, broccoli, eggs, some dairy, oats,
    cottage cheese, lentils, low-fat and low-sugar yoghurts, nuts
    and seeds, quinoa, whey protein supplements, wholegrain
    cereals, wholegrain pasta, wholegrain bread, all vegetables,
    potatoes with the skin on, salads without dressing but maybe a
    squeeze of lemon instead). Keep those up, but remember that
    is within the less food overall approach, so a higher proportion
    of those foods than others. A way of keeping good stuff good is
    to microwave, bake or grill it, not fry it.

4. Eat less of the bad stuff

    Keep the sugars, fats and alcohol down (fat strips on meat, pies,
    pastries, sauces, processed meat such as bacon, pizza, most
    take-away meals, chocolate, sweets, cakes, puddings, crisps,
    biscuits, sugary drinks including fruit juice). Notice how many
    of the better items (point 3) are natural products, and how
    many of the less-good items are processed.

5. Think about why you are eating and why.

    No more mindless eating because the TV is taking your
    attention rather than thinking about what you are consuming.
    Food and drink because you are diverted, or perhaps bored and
    a bit depressed, is a hidden menace, and guess what, boredom
    eating is always the less-good stuff. Calories for comfort is not
    a solution, physically or mentally. Food is not a hug.

6. Make wise choices when out

    Eating and drinking while outside your home needs thought.
    Try to make healthier choices and give the desserts and booze a
    miss if you can. If you can't cut out the booze, cut it down to
    one glass where otherwise you would have more. Fruit juice
    isn't a good substitute but iced, fizzy water with a slice of lemon
    is my choice.

7. Extra water is vital

    Talking of water, keep the water intake up throughout the day.
    The body needs it, it doesn't make you fat but does make you
    feel full and it's free. How good is that? And if it's boring, try it
    sparkling (sorry, it won't be free then) and chilled and with a
    slice of lemon or lime. You will want to drink at least two litres
    of water per day, some of which can be the water in whey
    protein shakes. Yes, it is possible to drink too much but most
    unlikely that you will.

8. Add more liquids

    Get extra hydration from additional sources. Tea and coffee are
    fine, but reduce the sugar and milk/cream, ideally to zero, as
    you have been heading towards already. Zero-calorie soft
    drinks are not really healthy but if you crave a diet soda, that's
    acceptable but no more than one can per day, as the
    sweeteners are seen by some as not being good for you. Also,
    remember caffeine can disrupt sleep so watch evening intake.

9. Morning cardio

    Try and do some exercise that raises the heart rate first thing in the morning. A brisk walk is fine and better if you can jog some of it. At least 20 minutes, 30 - 40 is better. Look to expend effort, not conserve it. Black tea or coffee before is helpful, but nothing else, except water of course. Then home to break your overnight fast with your break-fast.

10. Move more

    In addition to the morning cardio, find ways to incorporate movement into your life. Walk rather than drive or take the bus if it's not far. Always walk a little more quickly by pretending you are in a bit of a rush. Walk up any stairs rather than take the lift if it's only a few floors. Keep a look out for ways to spend additional energy through movement. Be creative: do you have loos both upstairs and downstairs at home? If so, always use the further one.

11. Get the muscles exercised

    Twice a week do some exercise at home: a warm up, some resistance exercises to work the key muscle groups, some work on the abdominals and a little stretching. Try and do ten repetitions of each movement. Once that is easy for any exercise, increase the number. Try to progress everything over time, either more repetitions, or a longer time, or heavier resistance. Note that doing an exercise slowly is better than doing it quickly, so slow down through all these.

    It could take only 15-20 minutes to do the full set but see if you can do each repetition more slowly to take longer. You can see and hear it in the video[18] specifically for this workout session and if you want to see this Stage One workout documented as well, that is in Appendix E.

12. Chill

Try to minimise stress in your life and get a good night's sleep. You've used extra energy in all that added movement and exercise and you've significantly improved your diet; and that should help with both of those.

As I said, only twelve guidelines but, as you see, there isn't much of your life than isn't affected by them. I don't think you'll remember everything in every item, but I hope the headline I've included for each point will help in recalling the details.

You don't have to follow all the guidelines all the time – but the more you stick to the guidelines and for more of the time, then the more likely you are to reach your target, and more quickly too. You knew that anyway but it doesn't hurt to reinforce the message. Read that sentence again (the one with all the 'all' words and even more 'more' words in it), and make sure the message gets stored in your long-term memory.

You don't need to remember anything else. Indeed, you don't need to read any more of this book until a week has passed since the Starting Date you wrote down. When you've reached that point, turn the page.

7 – The Weekly Stage One Review

Every week while you are on Stage One, I want you to return to the scales and note updated figures for your overall weight and bodyfat percentage. Do this at the same time of the time of day as the initial measurement, of course, and at exactly the same location and wearing the same, which is nothing.

Make a note somewhere of the figures and the date, then compare with the values you noted a week earlier. If this is your very first weekly review, then you'll be comparing with the starting numbers that you entered in Chapter 5.

One of several different things will have happened:

1. Your weight and bodyfat percentage have both gone down. Hooray, that's exactly what we wanted! Carry on as you have been for another week on Stage One. See you next week.

2. Your weight has gone down but not the bodyfat percentage. It is good news that you are losing bodyfat but not that you are losing muscle mass. In most cases this suggests you have reduced the quantity of food but the quality isn't where it should be. Remain in Stage One but put extra emphasis on eating fewer of the bad things (point 4) and more of the good things (point 3) and make sure you are drinking enough water. Feel free to add a few extra slow repetitions to the exercises too and maybe add a few minutes to your pre-breakfast cardio.

3. You bodyfat percentage has gone down but not your weight. This is very rare, but if it takes place it suggests you have lost bodyfat but added the same amount of muscle and water together, which is not altogether bad news! Remain in Stage One. You may be drinking too much water, so see if that condition continues for a second week.

4. Your weight and bodyfat percentage have both gone up. That's not what we wanted. It suggests you need to 'turn up the dial' on the twelve guidelines. Find ways to increase your level of adherence to the guidelines for next week. Remain in Stage One with the same guidelines, unless this is the second consecutive week that you are in this result of weight and bodyfat both increased. If that is the case, it's on to Stage Two from now with more details in the next chapter.

There is one other possibility: that you have reached your target weight and bodyfat numbers that you noted in Chapter 5. In other words, you are inside your Target Zone. This means success in a big way and I need a symbol to represent a high-five!

If that is you head now to Chapter 21. All good things come to an end so for you that is goodbye to Stage One and hello to Stage Three.

8 – Preparation for Stage Two

Stage Two is where you get rather more detailed in the approach to your fit-up and fat-down project.

To start with I'm going to suggest a few things that it would be good for you to acquire in order follow my Stage Two fitness recommendations I am mentioning these at the very beginning, so you can have them in place and 'hit the ground running' when you start on the Stage itself.

There are four of them and I believe the benefits you will derive from them and the progress they will help you to make will more than repay you. Don't think of these as costs, think of them as investments that will help you on your fitness journey. However, none of these four is mandatory and for each there is a lower-cost or zero-cost alternative. Those alternatives won't bring all the benefits of the actual item proposed in the same timescale, of course, and will doubtless involve you in more administrative tasks, but if you cannot justify the outlay then this is certainly better than dropping the idea of the fatness-down, fitness-up programme altogether.

Finally, on the money side, a side benefit is that if you have purchased what I suggest, then you are even less likely to decide that Stage Two is not for you. If you have already spent cash on this, you will want to stick around to see a return, won't you?

It could well be several days until you have everything ready for Stage Two, so carry on with the guidelines of Stage One until you are ready. Many a fitness project has been derailed before it really started by saying 'I'll start once I have got….' – a time which somehow never arrives.

Much of the enhanced measuring comes in the area of nutrition. You are going to start to count calories plus grams of four specific nutrients. But don't panic, these days this isn't a laborious task, not like when I did it a decade or so ago.

MyFitnessPal

This is smartphone app and a website that tracks your nutrition. It's easiest with a smartphone, as you can use the phone's camera to scan barcodes of food products. And with the phone, you have the app with you for use when you're not at home. But if you don't have one, then there is a web version.

Create an account with MyFitnessPal and enter your basic data on the Profile screen. Leave your nutrition goals for now, but you already have your current and target weight to enter and a rate of weight loss. Choose the option that you do not increase calories to be consumed as a result of exercise undertaken.

Notice how you can enter the food items you consume in the Diary function, adjusting the portion size as necessary. Many of the items you consume will already be stored in the large MyFitnessPal database and the ability to scan a barcode can save much time.

You don't need to start recording the foods you eat yet as that's covered in Chapter 12. At this stage, it's good that you are ready to go with MyFitnessPal.

If you're allergic to technology, then you can work with pen and paper to record this information but it's a big task and none of my clients, even the most technophobic, remained keen on pen-and-paper. They all came around to the MyFitnessPal approach, and now its second nature to them.

There is an extra-cost premium option on MyFitnessPal. It has features which are useful such as extra functionality to set nutrient targets in grams (rather than solely as a percentage) and removes adverts. I recommend that you select this option. It's worth having as you'll be using the app several times a day and anything that makes it easier to use is good. And you soon get fed-up with the adverts!

Smart Wearable Technology

In Stage Two, you will be counting your daily steps and comparing them against a target. There will be times when you are checking your heart rate and noting your daily calories of energy expended.

Technology comes to your assistance again here. The best way of achieving this is to wear a smartwatch, ideally the whole day long, charging it overnight. There are many models available and prices start much lower than you think. I've always been a fan of the Fitbit brand and I use a Versa3, but that's at the expensive end of the market.

Do a comparison of the features before you purchase one. The minimum functionality should be: time (of course, it is a watch!), heart rate, calories expended and steps taken per day.

There is always a doubt on the accuracy of these devices, and my view is that (1) each is accurate when compared to itself in terms of direction of travel. So, if it says you have burned more calories today than yesterday, than the direction is probably true even if not the exact numbers shown; and (2) it is far better than guesstimating.

An alternative is to use similar functionality on a mobile phone with apps as necessary. I don't recommend this as you may not have your phone with you all the time. It may be sitting on your desk as you walk around the office or home and I don't want you to take your phone into the weights area of the gym. The heart rate detection on a phone may require you to hold it in a certain way, which you can't easily do at all times, such as during a cardio session.

Create a Daily Data Sheet on Excel

It's good to monitor progress in a written way. Keeping a log of your key statistics is a major incentive to success – what gets written, gets done. Imagine this as a sheet of numbers in a table, one row for every day with various columns, and all those numbers going down the page indicate how successful you are being over time; a great motivation factor.

The best (but not the only) way of doing this is using Excel, and I'm assuming you have that available on a laptop or PC and are familiar with creating a simple spreadsheet. There's nothing complicated in the data recording and simple calculations I'm going to ask you to create, so advanced Excel knowledge is not required.

If you don't have Excel, then there are free spreadsheets for use on your phone. I use Utility Spreadsheet Pro from Luminant Software, and of course there are others. Finally, if you have no access or relevant skills in Excel or the phone, and if you don't want to move in that direction then a pen and paper will do fine, but again it's more work.

So, to your spreadsheet. You need to create a sheet with 15 columns. The first row is a header row, and the headers of each column to go into this first row are:

- Date, Weight, Weight-Ave, Bodyfat %, BF%-Ave, Kcal, Protein, Sugars, Fats, Sat Fat, Hours, Water, Cardio, Steps, Train.

The width of the data is for a date in the first column, then three digits for each of the net four columns and just one digit for each of the final ten columns. As part of the design, you can set the formats for the four columns for weight and bodyfat to be one decimal place, and the remaining columns to zero decimal places.

There will be one row per day going forwards. How far forward? Don't put a limit on it in your mind; it will be at least until you are in your Target Zone and by the time you get there, you'll probably want to continue. Put the first few dates in column one, but no more than that. Then save that as the Daily Data sheet. There is an example of the format in Appendix G.

I suspect you can already work out what is going to be stored in some of those columns from the headings I gave. You will find out if you are right, and see the meaning of the other columns, over the next few chapters and in Chapter 18.

If you are doubting the value of this Daily Data sheet, bear in mind that those people who keep written records of this type of data lose twice as much weight in total (or the same weight, twice as fast) as those that don't. That should be motivation indeed.

Gym Membership

I also want to move your twice-weekly workout to a gym and that's also the best place for your morning cardio too.

How to choose a gym? The obvious criterion is location. You'll be here most days of the week so make it easy to access, close to home or on your way to work. Hours of opening are important, and many UK gyms are now 24-hours (Anytime Fitness, Pure Gym, The Gym, for example).

Choose a gym that has a range of exercise machines, some free weights (dumbbells and benches) and also a cardio area that has running machines (treadmills) and cross-trainers (elliptical trainers), where you stand up and your feet move in pedalling motion with your hands-on long poles that move to assist the motion. If you're unsure which machines these are, check out my videos for treadmills[19] and cross-trainers.[20] That should help you identify them.

You will be spending significant time in the cardio area so you may want to ensure you can watch TV to keep your eyes busy during the exercise. All of the gyms from the national chains, including the three I've mentioned, should be fine on this and the other points I have mentioned.

See how busy the gym is typically at the hours you would normally attend, which ideally will be first thing in the morning for cardio and whenever you want later in the day to do a resistance training session. Most gyms are at their busiest between 5pm and 8pm weekdays, so check that time if you are concerned by how crowded it might be.

One of the most important things is not to be Gymtimidated. If you've read my story, you'll know this was a big factor for me, and I don't want it to be for you. Don't be dissuaded if you are the oldest person you can see, or the one that appears to be the least fit. Everyone was a newcomer to the gym once, your money is as good as anyone else's, and you should be proud of the fact that you are turning to the gym at your age – so many people don't do so. No one there is evaluating you and you aren't in competition with anyone at the gym. If you doubt any of this, ask any of the staff and they will tell you that they actively welcome people of our age group.

If you can't bring yourself to join a gym or if there isn't a convenient one, then you can continue the cardio as in Stage One. And for the twice-weekly weights workout, I have a no-gym workout you can follow, shown in Appendix H[21]. These are both less-than-perfect alternatives, but are far better than ignoring these aspects altogether.

Next Steps

I hope you are able to put those four preparatory steps in place. Assuming you have either done that, or are in the process of doing so, let me introduce you to the ten objectives in Stage Two.

9 – Stage Two: The Ten Objectives

As you know, Stage Two is where you become more detailed in the approach to your fatness-down and fitness-up project.

In summary, Stage Two formalises the guidelines of Stage One. There actually isn't anything much that is totally new; but the guidelines from Stage One have morphed into measurable objectives. A guideline is a suggested approach to something; turning it into an objective means that it can be measured – did you achieve the objective? And each such question has a simple Yes/No answer for each day.

I've mentioned more than once that 'what gets written, gets done'. Hence the need for recording progress on each objective every day. Much later we can review your Yes/No responses to individual objectives and use those to see which areas need more focus if you are not achieving your overall fit-up and fat-down targets.

There's more for you to do in this stage, compared to Stage One. More to be kept track of, more to be written. It's going to take more time. However, the approach used means the added time is kept to a minimum – especially after the initial set up is done. And you've taken the first, major, step in that set up already – acquiring the four pre-requisites in the last chapter.

It's important to note that you don't have to get a Yes result on every objective every day. The more Yes results you have per week the better, but you live in the real word and that just isn't going to happen. Bear in mind that the closer you get to a Yes on each one, the sooner you will reach your fit/fat targets. That's a vital point, and I wouldn't be surprised if I repeat it later.

1. Consume fewer calories per day than you expend.

2. Eat a substantial amount of protein.

3. Eat a limited amount of sugar.

4. Eat a limited amount of fat.

5. Within the fat that you consume, eat a limited amount of saturated fat.

6. Consume your calories over a set period of hours.

7. Drink a substantial amount of water.

8. Undertake some calorie-burning cardiovascular activity.

9. Move a minimum number of steps.

10. Perform some daily training – abs, stretching or weights.

Each of these objectives will be described in more detail in the chapters that follow. The concept is that, using the information in those chapters, you will be able to state either Yes or No as to whether you achieved that objective for a particular day. The more Yes results you get per week the better, and the sooner you will reach your goals.

For each objective that simple Yes/No test can be e recorded as a 1 for yes or a 0 for no. Any day when you achieved all ten would be recorded as a 1 1 1 1 1 1 1 1 1 1 – an amazingly good ten-out-of-ten day. And a day when you succeeded only the first and last objectives would be written as 1 0 0 0 0 0 0 0 0 1. Adding those 1's together, a perfect week would be 70 (I don't think you'll have many of those) and a rubbish week would total 0 (and I hope you don't have any of those). We are heading towards putting these 0 and 1 values into the relevant columns on the Daily Data sheet, in case you haven't guessed that already.

Before we do that, let's go into details on what you do to achieve success in each of these ten objectives. It's going to take some time to explain these, so carry on with the guidelines of Stage One until you are ready to cut over to Stage Two.

You may have noticed that the first five of the ten objectives are all connected with measuring the contents of your nutrition, more specifically the quality and amount of what you eat and drink. Chapters 11 and 12 explain this in more detail.

10 – Create Your TIC-TOC

What's this all about, then? I'm guessing that the last thing you need is another social media platform, especially one with a target market less than half your age.

Don't panic, it's something else entirely. It's all to do with calories, which is much more your cup of (sugar-free) tea, I know. It's a step in preparing for objectives 1-5 of Stage Two.

The first thing we will be looking at is redressing the balance of the Energy Equation or, more simply, using up more calories than we are consuming. It's this gap on which I want to focus. To lose weight we need to create a daily calorie deficit – where the number of calories you use exceeds your calories consumed. This is fundamental to losing weight. You won't lose weight on a daily calorie surplus.

There are a couple of steps to this. The first stage is to find a number for your calories used up by your typical day's activity. I call this your Typical Output Calories number – your TOC.

Most people burn around 50-80 calories an hour while lying in bed. Called the Basal Metabolic Rate, that's the energy used with the effort of breathing, keeping warm and all the body's internal processes that continue 24 hours a day. It's the movement you do on top of that: walking, moving your arms and head, even standing supporting your weight – plus exercise of course – that adds to the number. We are looking for your TOC, the total calories you use up on a typical day, the rest plus the active hours.

If you have a smartwatch, that probably gives you that number at the end of each day (if it doesn't, it isn't very smart). Find a recent day with typical levels of activity and take that figure. Or better, find a range of recent days and take the average. Obviously, don't take unusual days like ones where you slept most of the day due to illness, walked 20 miles or flew half-way around the world.

If you don't have a smartwatch, then your phone may give that information, although I have found phones are generally less good at keeping an accurate record. I mentioned one reason for this already: there is an assumption that you keep your phone in your pocket at all times. That's probably not the case; maybe it's on your desk and not with you as you move about, and also you may not have it when you are exercising or, of course, when it's getting charged.

Another option is to use a calories-used calculator like the one I have one[22] on my website. If you are using that tool, select 'moderate activity' if you have a sit-down job, or go for 'very active' if it's a walk-around job. That would also apply if you are going to be very enthusiastic about following my exercise advice, coming later.

Do you have your TOC? Excellent; that is the first stage done. That TOC is going to apply to you for the coming week. Every week you can review your TOC in the light of that week's activities, and adjust it if needed. There's more on that in Chapter 20 as we look at the Weekly Stage Two Review.

For the examples that follow, I'll use TOC of 2500 calories. Your number may be close to that, or higher or lower. Obviously use your number when calculating numbers for your own situation.

Now you have your TOC, you can work out your TIC, Target Input Calories, that is how many calories you aim to consume each day in the coming week. And that is determined by how much of a daily calorie shortfall you want to create.

Think about this table and select a rate you want to use:

Planned weight reduction per week – lb	Planned weight reduction per week – kg	Daily calorie deficit – TOC minus TIC
0.5	0.25	250
0.75	0.375	375
1	0.5	500
1.5	0.75	750
2	1	1000

Obviously, the further down the table you go, the quicker you will get results, but the harder it is to succeed. You may remember that the aim was to achieve a 1 lb (0.5 kg) per week weight reduction in Stage One. My generic suggestion is to try to accomplish that rate again here in Stage Two. You have the opportunity to review it weekly if that rate isn't working for you.

A simple subtraction will give you your daily target calories input, your TIC. I have selected the mid-point from this table as my example, an expected weight loss of 1lb or 0.5kg a week, so that's 500 to be subtracted from my TOC of 2500 giving a TIC of 2000. That's a convenient figure to use for the examples as 2000 is the calorie value used for the UK Government Reference Intakes of nutrients so you'll see it frequently on food nutrition labels.

Of course, your own calculation may well be different. Your own TOC minus your selected daily calorie deficit giving your TIC.

Any day where your calories consumed is at your TIC or a little below (up to say 10%) counts as that target having been achieved. I don't want you to consume too few calories so try not to end any day having consumed fewer calories than 90% of your TIC. You now have your Target Input Calories figure for every day in the coming week, which will be fundamental to your success in Stage Two.

Another key factor is the type and quality of food you eat. Even if you adhere to your TIC figure, you will look very different (and it will have a very different effect on your health) if those calories are all from broccoli, chicken or creamy jammy doughnuts.

There are some general principles about nutrition that are very helpful for you to understand at this point, both for your fat to fit journey and also for your health generally. I don't want to send you back to the classroom, but I suggest you review Chapter 3 if you need a reminder of these.

11 – Objectives 1-5: Nutrition

There are five elements of nutrition for which I want you to set targets and to track as part of Stage Two.

Those are firstly overall calories consumed, which we have already talked about, plus four values of weight of nutrients, each of which is measured by a daily total in grams, which you will be comparing to daily target values.

The complete list of five is:

- Total Calories
- Protein
- Sugar
- Fat
- Saturated Fat

The particularly good news is that MyFitnessPal will be doing a lot of the hard work for you such as all the additions and percentages. You do, however, have to set the target values and make the right choices when selecting your foods so that the numbers produced by MyFitnessPal are what you want them to be.

I've talked about the five nutrition things I want you to track on a daily basis: total calories, grams of protein, grams of sugar, grams of fats and grams of saturated fats. These are the five values I track in my own diet, of course.

The next stage is to add some real-world numbers target numbers to those five variables.

We are now going to set target daily values for the remaining four nutrition objectives. You should already have set the value for the first one, your target of calories consumed. It is your TIC value that you established in the last chapter.

The target values of the other four nutrition measures are all derived as a percentage of your TIC. You don't need to understand the maths involved in creating these percentage numbers as it is a little complicated. However, if you want to know more about these calculations turn to Appendix I for a detailed description.

- Protein is to have a target minimum value (in grams) of 7.5% of your TIC

- Sugar is to have a target maximum value (in grams) of 3.35% of your TIC

- Fat is to have a target maximum value (in grams) of 3.35% of your TIC

- Saturated Fat is to have a target maximum value (in grams) of 1% of your TIC

Here are the targets to be used for some typical TIC numbers:

Target Inwards Calories - TIC	Protein grams (min)	Sugar grams (max)	Fat grams (max)	Saturated Fat grams (max)
1600	120	53	53	16
1700	128	56	56	17
1800	135	60	60	18
1900	142	64	64	19
2000	150	67	67	20
2100	158	70	70	21
2200	165	73	73	22
2300	172	76	76	23
2400	180	80	80	24
2500	188	84	84	25
2600	195	87	87	26

Now work out your own target values for each of those four nutrients based on your own TIC, if it isn't one of the 11 shown above. You may want to write the numbers relevant to you below:

Target Inwards Calories - TIC	Protein grams (min)	Sugar grams (max)	Fat grams (max)	Saturated Fat grams (max)

Just to clarify – the number of grams for protein is a daily target minimum. For the other values, it is the daily target maximum.

12 – Recording the Nutrition

I'm going to ask you to log all the food and drink you consume. This was a really onerous thing to do in the old days, when I did it for my own weight loss, but these days technology has come to your rescue. The easiest way of keeping track of your nutrition is to use the MyFitnessPal app on your smartphone or PC. I'm going to assume that you have a smartphone and that you have installed and customised MyFitnessPal for your use as I described in Chapter 8.

Now would be a good time to enter your nutrition target numbers into the Goals section of MyFitnessPal. To do this:

1. Select More, then Goals, then 'Calorie, Carbs, Protein and Fat Goals'.

2. Input your TIC as the default goal for Calories.

3. Select 40% for Carbs, 30% for Protein and 30% for Fat. You should see the grams of protein and fat automatically calculated for you to be the grams from your table, above. Ignore the grams figure for Carbs. There is an explanation of the maths behind these percentage numbers in Appendix I, but this is complex and you don't need to know it.

4. Return to Goals and select 'Additional Nutrient Goals'. Input your grams figures for sugar and saturated fats. Other values can be left as the defaults shown.

5. You can check all the above by looking at the Diary screen – choose for tomorrow, then you may need to rotate the phone to landscape view to see Totals and Remaining.

6. You can choose the columns you want displayed here to be the ones we are tracking. This can't be done in the app but can be done on your account on MyFitnessPal.com. Go there then select My Home, Settings, Diary Settings; then under nutrients tracked, change to: Protein, Sugar, Fat, Saturated Fat.

7. Check the Diary setup again by looking at the Diary for tomorrow, rotating if required, and it should be set just right, with the correct nutrients being shown with your correct goal numbers.

You are now ready to start recording your food and drink in the Diary function. There are five numbers for you track, as you know: calories, protein, sugar, fat, saturated fat. Where do you find these numbers?

You know that for pre-packed food items, the numbers are on the nutrition label that legally has to be present. For these pre-packed items, MyFitnessPal is usually very good, and can be barcode scanned. Make sure that the volume is reasonable. If the numbers are for a 40g suggested portion size of a cereal, make sure that's the amount you are eating, and if it's not, adjust the number of portions. For example, if your cereal is 60g, you input that as 1.5 portions.

For non-pre-packed items that are shop-purchased, such as fresh meat and fish, loose fruit and vegetables, again you can find these numbers on MyFitnessPal in many cases. Factor the numbers due to the size, as no system knows how big your apple is. Either weigh it or make an honest assessment and adjust your numbers.

There's a bit of estimating going on there. That will become more important as we move on to eating food in a restaurant, take-away or at someone else's home.

If you are eating at a one of the big chains, then approximate values for many of the foods are on MyFitnessPal – I know that Harvester, Weatherspoon's and Pizza Express menu items are there as well as many others. These have to be approximate values as you don't know if they cooked with exactly the same amounts of ingredients that were used when the nutrition information was calculated.

If you are eating at a non-chain restaurant or at someone else's home, then one option is to compare with something that does exist on MyFitnessPal. For example: 'Well, I reckon this is probably equivalent to a Harvester 8oz Sirloin with Fries Meal' (which exists on MyFitnessPal). This also works with take-aways from small businesses, which won't be on MyFitnessPal. There are values for most generic items that you can use if it's close to an equivalent item.

Finally, if all else fails, break down the meal into its component parts and evaluate each separately. That's not an easy task and one that could easily destroy the romance of a candlelit meal à deux, I suspect; unless your partner is impressed by your plans to improve your fitness, of course.

Whatever you do and whatever you eat, no matter how big or small, don't just ignore it. An estimation of values is better than no figures just because you think you may not be close. Just make sure you are being realistic and not rounding down every time. Over time you will get good at estimating; I did.

There's a drawback to the program that I sometimes see. For some food items MyFitnessPal will give an overall calorie value, but no nutrient information. You won't see the protein, sugar, fats, saturated fats or any other component of those calories. Keep an eye out for that, and select (or create) a different food item instead.

A slight diversion: Back in the days when I had a real job, I worked in IT systems for banks. I've seen some good ones and some poor ones. The very worst systems are input-only processes, where people enter data into a computer and the system stores it, but it is never accessed to provide useful information. If it is ever output, nobody ever looks at it, or if they do, they never act on it. That was more than a decade ago. There aren't any processes left where that still applies, surely? (You bet there are!).

Why I am describing this? Because, so far, I have described MyFitnessPal is an input-only system. Of course, I want you to look at the results from it, and use that to guide your future behaviour. As you enter the day's food and drink into the Diary screen, check the totals of the five variables at the bottom. You may need to rotate the screen to landscape view to see it; and if it is showing percentages, tap the top row to change to grams.

The usual approach to MyFitnessPal is to enter each food and drink item as you consume it or soon afterwards, in the way I've described above. You're unlikely to forget anything if you do it 'enter-as-you-eat' during the day. The drawback is that you can't see where the numbers are heading for by the end of day. Have you left enough calories for dinner and are you going to be under on protein or over on sugar?

The better way to use the app is by entering your predicted food and drink for that day into the Diary function first thing in the morning. Plan what you will be eating and when. Input that information as if it had already taken place. Review what the totals are predicted to be at the end of the day, and then go back and make the changes you want to your planned day's eating and drinking. Once you're happy, you've done a great job at planning your eating for the day ahead. You are far less likely to deviate from the plan for that day as that plan has now been created (by you) and you now 'own' that day's plan. Time for another of my favourite fitness phrases: 'Plan your eats, then eat your plan'.

This becomes easier once you have done at least a few days of enter-as-you-eat. That's because you can scan an item's barcode the first time you encounter it. It then will come up as a suggestion next time you type in a few characters, which makes it easier for this morning-data-entry predictive approach for items you have eaten before.

One of the good points of using the app in this 'predict-the-day' way is that you can update your day in MyFitnessPal as it proceeds. Perhaps things change and you eat differently from your plan. You can go back into the Diary, replace the planned data item with the actual, and again see the day's forecast totals and make any adjustments necessary to your plan for the rest of the day.

If you haven't already started, now would be a good time to 'go live' with using MyFitnessPal. Enter what you have eaten so far today, and then forecast what you will be consuming for the rest of the day.

To try out a full day, input what you think you will eat tomorrow. Take a guess if you don't really know – you can always change later. Check the totals and adjust as necessary to make it a good day on your nutrition numbers. Do you notice a feeling of you being in control of your eating, rather than your eating being in control of you, while entering these in-advance, projected meals?

Now you have tomorrow already set down in writing, it will be much easier to hit those targets when tomorrow comes. You just follow your plan. Plan your eats, then eat your plan.

If you are using MyFitnessPal as-you-go, rather than predictive, you obviously can't actually change what you've eaten already that day. Even so, it can help you make choices for the remainder of the day. Try going predictive after a few days.

You are starting to use MyFitnessPal as the fundamental tool to help you succeed in Stage Two. Does it seem to take a long time? You'll find the time drops rapidly as you become used to it. I do exactly what I'm asking you to do and it takes me less only a couple of minutes of my time per day, now I am used to doing it. I suspect you will find the same.

Successful use of MyFitnessPal will lead to achieving 50% of your daily Stage Two objectives because it's the first five of the ten daily objectives. As I am sure you have deduced by now, you'll be updating your Daily Data sheet by putting a 1 for each objective that you achieved on a specified date, and a 0 if you didn't. Use the columns labelled Kcal, Protein, Sugar, Fat and Sat Fat.

You can do that entry of those five zeros or ones for the completed day either now or later. You can enter those for all ten objectives any time after you have finished eating and drinking for the day. That works, but you may want to wait until first thing tomorrow so that you can enter for the other five objectives, updating the sheet at one time early tomorrow for all ten objectives for today. There's more about updating the Daily Data sheet, including how and when, in Chapter 18.

13 – Objective 6: Hours

A key way to help the body to use more bodyfat as fuel is to give it no alternative. And the best and easiest way to do this is to maximise what is already the body's longest fat-burning period: overnight, starting from a few hours after your last meal.

Put very simply, the body will use the fuel from whatever you have eaten to fuel itself for the next few hours. That's how most of the day goes by. You don't usually eat overnight, but the body still needs fuel for keeping you alive and the repair and maintenance tasks. So, the body will use the fuel in your last evening's consumed calories for the first part of overnight, then will turn to its built-in reserve for the next few hours. That built-in fuel reserve is your bodyfat, which is of course previously consumed fuel that you haven't used yet.

The body will use that fuel source – provided you don't do any strenuous exercise – right up until you ingest some calories of food or drink again in the morning. So, prolonging this no-food period significantly helps by making the body turn to its fat reserves for fuel. That switch, from using accumulated sugars as fuel to using bodyfat is called 'metabolic switching' and of course, once you eat and start to digest the switch moves in the other direction.

The easiest trick I know to keep the switch in the 'burn-bodyfat' setting is to have a 12-hour period every day (which is overnight) without eating. So, if your last calories inwards were at 9pm, don't have anything else until 9am. If you are out late and eating until 11pm, then tomorrow's breakfast is at 11am. And if you know you have to have breakfast at 7am tomorrow then plan to eat no later than 7pm today.

It's that simple. The overnight no-eating period is, of course, a fast – hence the name for your morning meal, break-fast.

To make this more effective, try to have some cardiovascular exercise early in the morning before the end of the 12-hour fast, and that's coming in the next chapter. One tip I'll mention here and again in that chapter: maybe have some black coffee before that exercise session. It stimulates the metabolism, helps the calorie-burn rate and also opens up the fat cells and encourages the release of fat to the bloodstream for use as fuel.

By the way, that black coffee is allowed in the 12-hour non-eating period as it has no calories. Water and black or herbal tea are the same; they are allowed as they have no calories. So, the idea is not specifically avoiding anything in that fasting period, it's keeping clear of calories.

If you enjoy your overnight fast, you could grow it to 14 or 16 hours, but don't be tempted to extend it beyond that as this can have the opposite effect. A long fast can put the body into what is known as the State of Alert and elicits the Starvation response, with the body going all unwell on you and clinging on to bodyfat, as it thinks times have gone really tough and no food is coming for goodness-knows how long.

If you achieved a 12-hour period with no inwards calories overnight, you will enter a 1 for today under the Hours column when you have your Daily Data spreadsheet open. If you didn't achieve that, you should enter a 0.

14 – Objective 7: Cardio

Cardio activity, also called CV, is short for cardiovascular. This is the type of exercise designed specifically to improve endurance, to improve the body's aerobic system and by far its most popular use, to burn bodyfat.

Actually (and this really isn't important at all) I have never understood the term 'cardiovascular'. Cardio means to do with the heart and vascular means to do with the blood, and since blood is to do with the heart, that's a bit of duplication. I would prefer 'cardiorespiratory' – abbreviated to CR – to show that it is to do with both the heart and breathing hard, using the lungs in addition to the blood/heart. I realise I'm not going to change the language single-handedly, so I'll stop being pedantic and will just call it cardio, as most people do.

The objective here is to perform a single period of substantial amount of cardio exercise every day. By substantial I mean something that will burn several hundred calories in one go. I'm not going to set a target for calories burned here, as there are so many variables – type of cardio, speed, your weight, any added resistance and your heart rate are just the first few that come to mind. However, in most people I would expect it to be at least 30 minutes duration, or building up to that over time.

Monitoring your cardio is based on heart rate beats per minute (bpm), which indicate how intense an exercise is. Intensity can be measured by the percentage of a person's theoretical maximum heart rate being used during an exercise. Opinions and calculation methods of maximum rate vary, with the simplest calculation of that theoretical maximum number being 220 minus your age.

Most sources agree that the fat-burning zone of the body is when the heart rate is between 70% and 80% of that theoretical maximum. As a result, for a typical 55-year-old, the target cardio heart rate is usually between 116 and 132 bpm. I would suggest using a mid-point, 75% of maximum, at 124, all other factors being ignored. Start lower than this if you are unsure of your ability here, and definitely at a low rate if you have no means of measuring your heart rate.

Why don't I suggest cardio at higher-intensity number throughout, say at 85% or more? After all, more energy (calories) would be used? The reason is that at higher percentages the body tends to use a greater proportion of muscle mass as fuel and a lower proportion of bodyfat; you are trying to lose bodyfat here, not muscle. And, at the other end of the scale, too much at a low intensity means there's scope for harder work to be undertaken to achieve greater bodyfat utilisation. Not many fat-sourced calories would be utilised for the time involved if working steadily at a low intensity.

It's key to be able to monitor your heart rate for all types of cardio. Yours is probably shown on your smart watch, and if you don't have one, then your phone perhaps displays it. Some cardio equipment has this functionality built in, although ease of use varies. It's easy to hold the heart rate sensors on a cross-trainer, for example, and difficult (indeed, not recommended) while on a treadmill.

There are at least two theories on fat burning and cardio. They both work, one may be better than the other for any individual but I will cover the two of them so that you can choose either or maybe alternate between approaches, which is what I do. I call these HIT and MISS workouts. HIT is my slight abbreviation of HIIT – High-Intensity Interval Training. I shortened it by one 'I' to make it easier to pronounce, and so it goes nicely with MISS, which is training at Medium-Intensity Steady State.

Now I'll describe the two types, starting with MISS, the easier one to explain.

<u>MISS cardio</u>

I find the cross-trainer[23] is the ideal equipment for this, and most of my clients agree. It's easy to adjust the resistance and speed, and also to monitor heart rate. It doesn't require concentration all the time; you can probably watch TV or listen to music at the same time for most of the 30 minutes. By the way, I enjoy MISS so much, I do 40 minutes – but you can do 30!

The objective is to keep your heart rate at a steady state through this medium intensity exercise, that steady state being 75% of your theoretical maximum heart rate. Since it's impossible to keep to an exact number, I suggest you try to maintain the rate within 2 bpm above or below the rate given by that 75% number. To save constantly adjusting the resistance, I suggest you check only on the exact minute and change then. As with all cardio, it will take a little time for your heart rate to get up to speed, of course. Just working harder doesn't bring an instant response in heart rate.

It's fine if you prefer other items of cardio for your 30 minutes of 75% maximum:

- Walking fast/jogging/running on the treadmill[24] works well, but it is quite hard on the knees if you are not used to it, whereas the cross-trainer softens knee impact. Typically, the calories per minute are higher on treadmill than the on the cross-trainer, especially at faster speeds.

- Rowing and the stair-climber are both good, but I find the heart rate gets into the over-80% zone very quickly, and I have to proceed irritatingly slowly; you may find otherwise. Some people (like me) find the rowing machine generates pain in the lower back over time so I avoid for it for that reason too. Again, you may find otherwise.

- I think the stationary bike is in general just a bit too easy and not giving enough return for your time, probably because the body is supported and stationary. You don't derive the most energy-used-per-minute from it compared to other cardio options due to sitting down all the time. If you have excess bodyweight, that means there are extra kilos to be used as additional weight to be moved in a cardio exercise, and being seated doesn't use that mass to your calorie-burning advantage.

If you are not a member of a gym, then you are probably limited to the first one: walking, building up over time into a jog and eventually a run; but beware both of the trip hazards out on the street or park, and the pavement is less forgiving on knees than the gym treadmill. I wouldn't recommend cycling in the street as a form of heart rate determined cardio as managing relations with other traffic and road conditions while moving at a speed to create a high heart rate is not always easy.

If you are a fan of parkrun on Saturdays, which I hope you will be one day, then that activity counts as the cardio for that day.

HIT Cardio

This is more complex and I suggest you have at least a few days on the MISS approach before trying it. It is best to be comfortable with the controls of the machines, monitoring heart rate and using your displayed heart rate as a guide to effort before adding the innovations that HIT brings. I'll describe it using the treadmill as that's the ideal cardio equipment for HIT.

If you are ready to be HIT with the details, here are the key differences from MISS. Theory first: HIT cycles the heart rate up and down – from high heart rate to low heart rate and back again, and does this repeatedly for the full 30-minute duration. The concept behind HIT is that calories are burnt based on two factors: (1) the actual work being performed and (2) the heart rate. For the first, there's no real way to do more work without, erm, doing more work. So, the additional part of this theory concentrates on the second part, where you can benefit from excess calorie use without doing extra work, but from manipulation of the heart rate.

More detail: As you start performing extra work (such as going from walking slowly to running quickly) then the heart rate rises accordingly; it rises relatively quickly. Once you stop running, the heart rate slows down to the resting rate, but it does this return to a slower rate much more slowly. This excess burn as it slows down post-exercise is the higher heart rate that leads to the extra calorie use. Ten seconds after switching from a fast run to a slow walk, you aren't burning many calories from the current exercise, but your heart rate is still high, so the body is burning extra calories without doing the work to cause that higher rate. Result, more calories are burnt than the exercise speed would suggest.

To make this effective over time, you repeat the process. A series of intervals is created: run fast for two minutes, heart rate rises quickly to match it, then walk slowly, heart rate drops slowly and keep on walking until heart rate is down to 65% of theoretical maximum, then start again. By repeating these intervals, a number of these periods where you are burning excess calories without working for it are achieved.

Conclusion

As mentioned in the last chapter and without doubt, the best time for your cardio is first thing in the morning before consuming any calories. This maximises the body-fat burning potential of the exercise as well as giving you something to do (other than eat) in the final hour or so of your overnight fast.

If your personal domestic timing doesn't allow that, then any time during the day is fine, with the longer gap after food the better. Cardio an hour after food is good, three hours after food is better.

I don't advise cardio in the evening. Your heart rate is likely to remain high for some time after the exercise and trying to sleep with an elevated heart rate is tough. You will want to do some other training though, perhaps in the evening, as described in Chapter 17.

It is vital to remain well-hydrated during your cardio. That pre-exercise black coffee doesn't count as sufficient hydration for early morning cardio! I drink 0.5 litre (one pint) of water spread across the period before, during and immediately after the cardio session, and the same again with my breakfast, soon afterwards. You should plan on something similar. I'll talk more about hydration next.

See Appendix B If you are interested in more details of how I perform my HIT and MISS cardio sessions at an even greater level of detail.

If you achieved at least a single, continuous 30-minute cardio session during the day (I won't hold you to the early-morning time-slot) then enter a 1 for today under the Cardio column when you have your Daily Data spreadsheet open. If you didn't achieve that, you should enter a 0.

15 – Objective 8: Water

I'm sure you know this already but water is used for literally hundreds of tasks inside the body. Around 50-60% of the body's weight is water, and there's hardly any process within the body that isn't made worse though insufficient hydration levels.

This is even more the case while you are on a fit-up, fat-down plan. Muscles thrive on water; indeed, they are composed of water (well, almost, 80% of muscle is water) and even a small deficit can lead to muscles becoming ineffective and weaker.

Apologies in advance to vegetarians for this imagery, but think of a juicy, fresh uncooked lean cut of steak with the water within it keeping it that way. Put it under the grill for too long and all the liquid has gone. It's shrivelled up, smaller, lighter and less pliable. There's your dehydrated muscle – ineffective and unhealthy.

Bodyfat, on the other hand, doesn't absorb much water. Another food analogy – pour some water on a slab of butter and watch it lie on top. Your bodyfat, like butter, does not absorb water. As your percentage of bodyfat decreases, your percentage of water increases – because either you have more water-absorbing muscle than before, or you have lost less muscle compared to the bodyfat lost.

It is likely that your bioelectrical impedance scales can measure your hydration. It's not part of the Fat to Fit at Fifty plan to track this but you certainly can do so if you wish. I find there's almost always a perfect correlation – bodyfat percentage goes down, water percentage increases. That's a two-way relationship; by increasing your water, you are likely to preserve and add to muscle mass and bodyfat percentage goes down. You may want to check it every few months to ensure it is heading in the right direction. And if you find your water percentage is less than 45% for females and 50% for males, take a trip to your GP.

Your water needs are going to grow while you are getting fitter. You are moving more and that's extra water in exhaled breath and of course more sweating. You'll be placing more demands on your muscles. More muscle means more intramuscular water.

Another benefit of increased water consumed is that water in your stomach makes you feel fuller. You are less likely to want to grab some unneeded snack calories.

To make all this work, you have to drink water. I predict it will be more than you're drinking already, perhaps a lot more. A typical approach often used is to drink when you are thirsty; that doesn't work so well past the age of fifty. The body's internal messaging works a bit less efficiently at our age, so don't count on waiting until you have that level of thirst before reaching for the water.

Water in protein shakes counts, by the way, although the jury is out on whether coffee, tea or diet cola qualifies. My vote is no, since there's caffeine in there that acts as a diuretic, something that speeds the flow of water through the body. Also, alcohol – which I know you are minimising anyway – definitely doesn't count.

So how much water? An approach that works for me and that I recommend to others is 0.5 litre at the start of each 3-hour block of the 12-hour eating day, and one at the end too – so that's 2.5 litres in total. By the way, if you're old school, half a litre is a pint glass filled 90%.

The timing is up to you, but here are some suggestions:

- I advise that the first 0.5 litre is spread across before/during/ after morning cardio and I see that as essential. You shouldn't do serious cardio without serious hydration. Add an extra 0.5 litre if you are still keen to drink at the end, especially if you have sweated substantially.

- The second I usually recommend is the protein shake you may have with breakfast, soon after the cardio.

- The third is around lunchtime, the fourth in the afternoon and the fifth early evening. The third, fourth or fifth could be another protein shake after the weight training session if one is scheduled for that day.

The water taken with the cardio and the two as shakes are consumed fairly quickly. For the other two, don't drink 0.5 litre in one go, rather sip and spread it across the time up until the next one is due. Females need a little less, so if you are following that kind of timed approach, fill the glass or bottle about 75% each time.

Finally, it is possible to drink too much water, but most unlikely that you will do so with these activity and amount guidelines.

The measure of success on this is very subjective. It is simply, have you had a significant amount of water that day?   I don't want to ask you to count or measure more variables, but if you need a value on 'significant', I would go for that 2.5 litres for a male and about 2 for a female; and of course, more if you feel thirsty.

If you achieved that, then enter a 1 for today under the Water column when you have your Daily Data spreadsheet open. If you didn't achieve that, you should enter a 0.

16 – Objective 9: Steps

The daily cardio exercise I described in Chapter 14 is a substantial contributor to your daily calorie burn. That is the main reason you are doing it.

However, it doesn't necessarily burn the greatest number of calories over the course of your day. You can burn many more and further improve your health and fitness by moving generally more than you have up to now. Obviously, the calorie burn rate is lower during your walking around during the day than in the cardio, but the many extra hours you have outside of the cardio activity make just walking around as part of your daily life a real NEAT calorie burner.

NEAT is a term used in health and fitness, and stands for Non-Exercise Activity Thermogenesis. That last word means the production of heat in the body, which you can treat as the burning of calories; and the first bit relates to this not being part of your exercise or sport; in other words, calories used in your normal non-exercise activity. Primarily walking, but lifting, sweeping, ironing, washing, gardening, cleaning and 101 other things. Sitting in a car or on a sofa are not big contributors to NEAT, of course.

It is easily possible to burn twice or three times the calories you've used in the cardio in this NEAT way; and all you have to do is keep your non-exercise activity up. This was easier in the days when we all had manual jobs in fields or heavy jobs in industry, and we probably walked to and from the workplace too. Lots of energy was used there. These days many people have office jobs which involve hours of sitting and perhaps drive there from home.

Perhaps you can see why modern life is creating an environment where more people store bodyfat than before, and don't get me started on the added-calorie effect of fast food which can even be delivered to your door. This environment we have created for ourselves is called obesogenic – meaning a tendency to create obesity in the population, as a result of moving less and eating more less-healthful foods. What we are doing here in Fat to Fit at Fifty is backtracking to a time when this tendency so wasn't quite so prevalent.

I'm getting side-tracked here. Because of the non-manual labour jobs that many of us have and the labour-saving devices that we own, it has been estimated that the NEAT for an average person in the West can be 50% of what it was fifty years ago, and 25% of what it was a hundred years ago.

This is leading to my suggestion that you look for opportunities to move wherever you can in the majority of your life that isn't exercise. Walk rather than drive or take the bus if it's not far. Whenever you are walking, try walking more quickly than you have been used to. You will find your heart rate increases, you breathe more deeply, you probably move your arms and upper body more, all as well as taking bigger and/or more steps. All of these contribute to a greater rate of calorie burn. If you walk 30% faster than before then you will burn around 30% more calories per hour. Furthermore, most people feel better mentally after a fast walk when compared to dawdling. So, it is great exercise, contributes to your fat loss, is good for your overall physical and mental health, costs nothing and you get to where you were going sooner than you would have done, therefore giving you more time to do whatever it is you were going to do when you got there. Where is the downside in any of that?

Stairs are another great source extra calorie burn. Walk up any stairs rather than take the lift if it's only a few floors. I have a notional figure of four floors and if it's more than that, I take the lift; less than that, I walk. On the subject of stairs, walk up them two at a time if you can. It's a little bit of extra cardio, it's a short workout developing strength and flexibility for your legs and core, and you probably reach the top quicker. Another tip on stairs: do you have loos both upstairs and downstairs at home? If so, always use the further one.

Ever go on an escalator? Walk up and down them rather than ride. You burn calories and save time that way, maybe catching an earlier train as a result.

There's one extra point to be considered by those who sit working at a screen or watch TV for hours. Every hour, get up and walk briskly to somewhere that is two or three minutes away. Ideally, you'll arrive at somewhere you can have some water. Then walk back. Stand up straight while walking because your posture could probably do with a bit of correction after having been seated for so long. It would be good not to look at a screen for those five minutes, which includes not looking at your phone. Your eyes will thank you too, especially if you can go outside or look through a window at some distant things. If you regularly become so occupied you would miss the time, timers and apps are available that can be set to beep at hourly intervals.

So, how do we measure all this NEAT stuff? Any movement will burn calories of course and that will be reflected in your increased calories used during the day. More than that, we can be more specific than that on the steps taken, as that can be measured. All you have to do is count your steps over the day.

You don't have to count the steps yourself, of course. A device will do it for you. Your smartwatch is best, your phone will probably also work, but obviously your phone won't count any steps when it isn't with you.

How many steps? The simple answer is more than you have been doing so far, by perhaps 20%. Look at a day with typical levels of activity, and take that figure. Or, better, find a range of recent days and take the average. Obviously, just as when you were determining your typical calorie burn, don't take unusual days like ones where you slept most of the day due to illness, walked 20 miles or flew half-way around the world. Start from an average day and add that 20% to set yourself a target.

If you prefer to be allocated a number target rather than base it on your own activity, go for 12,000 per day. If you find you can achieve that number most days without increasing your activity then make it 15,000. If those seem like huge numbers, remember your daily cardio is included. Most smartwatches and phones include in their logging process the steps taken on the elliptical movement of a cross-trainer as well as those walked, jogged or run in their logging process, as the motion is similar enough. It is likely you will have already logged a few thousand steps from that, ideally before breakfast. Then you can have a highly NEAT day to follow.

If your step-counter shows you achieved your target, then enter a 1 for today under the Steps column when you have your Daily Data spreadsheet open. If you didn't achieve that, you should enter a 0.

17 – Objective 10: Training

This is final objective of the ten and, as sometimes happens, the one with the most detail. But since you've made it this far, I'm sure you can follow this one too.

The objective is 'training'. Obviously, the daily cardio plus the steps (described in Chapters 14 and 16) are major contributors to the additional calorie burn you are looking to achieve to help in the fit-up, fat-down project. They count as a part of your daily exercise.

However, there are more types of exercise that are beneficial to you, ones which should also form part of your activity. These exercise types are less focussed specifically on calorie burn, more on other body benefits which improve both your fitness in the short term and are longer-term preparation for you to take on the years ahead in an independent and confident way.

The three areas I want you to include in this objective are:

- Weight training with the objective of minimising the loss of muscle that occurs during a period of overall bodyweight loss. Ideally this is not just minimising loss but actually maintaining or even increasing muscle mass slightly, with the aim of combating frailty and strength loss.

- Core strengthening and stabilising, through a group of exercises dedicated to developing and reinforcing your mid-section – that's the abdominals (abs) and neighbouring muscles.

- Stretches to improve your flexibility, mobility, balance and co-ordination.

One of these training sessions can be undertaken per day, trying to keep an even spread across the week. A perfect week will therefore have two training sessions from any two from the above list, and three sessions of the third. Don't perform the same type of training on two adjacent days; if it was Core training on Monday, then perform the Stretching training or Weight training on Tuesday. You choose how to split it across the week.

You can perform these training sessions on the same day as your cardio, but leave a decent gap between them, at least six hours. If you are doing your cardio first thing in the morning, make the weights, stretching or core training session that afternoon or evening.

Before you start on anything described in this chapter, please re-read the advice on suitability of exercise for you as an individual in Chapter 1. In summary don't take on anything that gives you concerns without discussing it first with your GP or a qualified Personal Trainer at your gym.

I'll describe each of these three types of session:

Weight Training Session

This is the most complex of the three training sessions. It is also the longest in duration, taking around 40 minutes.

It also takes much longer to describe. One of the reasons for that is that people of fifty-plus often need more convincing to undertake a weights training session rather than core or stretching. I wish that were not the case because they are all equally important as the years progress.

This session is best performed in a gym, unlike the core and stretching sessions which are equally effective if undertaken at home. If you don't have access to a gym, then there is a no-gym alternative in Appendix H which actually combines the weights and core sessions into one single session. It is rather less effective than following the separate full gym and core routines below but far better than missing either aspect, and more advanced than the simple home-based workout suggested back in Stage One.

Welcome to the weights area of the gym, where all the strange-looking machines, free weights, benches and mirrors are. At first this will seem like an unusual world, one that you will make you doubt whether you belong here. It felt like that to me on my first visit with everyone else half my age and already twice as fit. You can overcome this; if you have any doubts re-read my comments on gym membership in Chapter 8.

Assuming you're now happy here, let's think about why you are here. No, it's not just because I suggested it. You're not here to become a champion weightlifter or bodybuilder, but to make progress with your fitness-up and fatness-down aims. And to help in doing that, you are going to work on some muscles. Why will that help?

Firstly, we are taking on our old adversary, sarcopenia. You may remember back in Chapter 1, I described this condition as being the natural loss of muscle mass and muscle function as we age, making us weaker and more frail with the passing years. You can't cancel sarcopenia, but a maintained or increased muscle mass level is a key contributor to delaying it.

Adding muscular strength will help you in everyday activities too, which will become more noticeable as you age. My gran couldn't pick up a heavy saucepan and, more seriously, when she fell, she didn't have the strength to push herself back up. A more trivial example: have you ever had to help someone older than you put a bag into an aircraft overhead locker and retrieve it afterwards? Ignoring the fact that it was too heavy anyway and should probably have gone in the hold, it is your chest and triceps muscles that you are using for wedging it in, and your back and biceps for heaving it out.

Muscle is more metabolically active than bodyfat. Every pound of muscle on your frame burns around eight calories a day, which is about four times the rate of a pound of bodyfat. This is because muscle has to be kept warm and supplied with blood and water, whereas bodyfat just sits there, needing far fewer resources from the body. As a result, owning muscle actually helps you with calorie burn.

One other relevant point is that muscle takes up less space than fat - about 20% less volume for the same weight. So, your overall size will be less for every pound of fat that you lose and replace with muscle. You will look trimmer, which is definitely one of your aims.

Many people say they don't want more muscle mass; they just want to be toned. I have news for you: there isn't any such thing as toning a muscle. Instead, you have to work on the shape of the muscle by gym training and also reduce the layer of bodyfat surrounding it. Those two steps together are what is meant by the term 'toning'.

I hope I've convinced you to start on the weights. If yes, the next question. How do you convert bodyfat to muscle?

Sorry, you can't. You can reduce bodyfat, and you can add muscle, but those are two totally separate body processes. You can't change one into the other. That works in the other direction too. If you ever hear anybody say that all their muscle has turned to fat, it absolutely hasn't.

Adding muscle is much harder than losing bodyfat. Just maintaining the same amount of muscle is a real victory. In order to maintain it you have to add back the muscle lost in your calorie-deficit life or limit its loss. During a lower-calorie phase, the default situation is that the body loses mass at an equal rate between muscle (which includes lots of water) and fat.

Taking an overly simple example, say you are 80kg overall with 30% of that fat and 70% muscle, ignoring the weight of bones, organs etc. If you lose 10kg and retain the same percentages, which is the likely result of a default weight loss approach, you will have lost 3kg of fat (from

24kg to 21kg) and 7kg of muscle (from 56kg to 49kg). You are 10kg lighter, still with the same bodyfat percentage, but you've lost a lot of muscle along with the excellent loss in bodyfat. But this isn't what we want. Had you lost the same 3kg of fat but not gained or lost any muscle, that makes you 77kg, with your bodyfat percentage dropping to 27% and your muscle percentage growing accordingly. Definitely a better result for future fitness.

We are able to maintain this muscle during a weight-loss phase using a combination of things we have already talked about: calorie deficit, additional hydration to keep muscles healthy, and increased levels of protein to build and maintain muscle mass – plus the new benefits from this section, which is resistance training.

Weight training, also called resistance training, is why I'm asking you to head to the weights area of the gym two or three times a week. On each visit I want you to work on the key muscle groups in the body. I suggest you perform exercises that are targeted at specific body parts. That way you can track how each body part is progressing, perhaps getting stronger over time.

The principle I advise is called incremental progressive overload. Muscles develop through being stimulated and made to work harder by moving a resistance that is being incrementally and progressively increased over time. There are a number of rules and suggestions for you to follow. I am sorry about the rules because I don't like rules, but I want this to be a beneficial gym visit for you, not one where there is an increased risk of injury, so rules are rules, and here they are:

1. Leave behind rings, bracelets, necklaces and anything else that can get caught. Take a sweat towel with you, and some water.

2. Before starting any exercise, study what is involved and how to do it. In particular note which body parts are meant to move and which are not. Check my videos, or ask, if you want to see

how an exercise is performed. Other people working out will be happy to help (but don't ask if they are mid-exercise!) and staff members there are of course being paid to help you.

3. If you are about to use a machine read the instructions and make sure you are at the correct seat settings, height etc. Use any safety features provided, such as the stop setting on the Smith Machine or Leg Presses, and ask anyone to 'spot' you if you are unsure of any free weight exercise and feel that dropping it could lead to a bad outcome. People rarely say no.

4. Choose a weight that is within your capabilities for the first time you ever perform an exercise; you will need to experiment to find this. You need to be able to do a set of ten continuous repetitions in good form as described next. A repetition, or rep, is a single movement of the resistance to its maximum extent then back to the starting position. And a set is a continuous group of reps.

5. Good form is of paramount importance. This means only moving those body parts that are meant to move for the exercise. Should you find yourself moving any other body part, at best it is cheating and reducing the effectiveness of the movement and at worst it is tempting injury. Count the reps, and make the reps count.

6. Do things slowly. Each rep should be about three to five seconds. In particular control the lowering phase, so resist gravity and don't let the weight drop and suddenly stop the movement at the lowest point. Again, that would be reducing effectiveness and promoting injury. Lower slower.

7. Don't hold your breath at any point. If you want to practise the most effective breathing technique, breathe out as you push or

pull against the resistance, breathe in as you resist gravity and lower slower. I call this Exonex – Exhale on exertion.

8. Try to avoid locking out the arms or legs. If you do, your skeleton is taking the weight, not the muscle, and that does nothing helpful in the muscle department. Stop the motion just short of lock-out to ensure this doesn't happen.

9. Start your workout with a set designed as a warm-up. Go through a full range of movement from your planned first exercise but with a lower resistance and a faster pace. Maybe half the resistance, twice the reps (therefore 20).

10. When you've finished an exercise, put away any dumbbells and tidy away any other free weights. Wipe down surfaces you've touched so they are ready for the next user. And take a sip of water, more if needed.

Those rules apply to whatever you do in the weights area of the gym now or in the future and not just my suggested workout, of course.

Now let's move from rules to the guidelines of the workout I suggest for you. First, here is a table of exercises. I would like you to perform one exercise from each row. You choose which one.

All exercises shown are safe but only if performed correctly and within your capabilities. Many newcomers prefer machines rather than free weights as, generally speaking, there is less likelihood of injury if there's a problem. I've put those in the first column.

Videos[25] exist for all exercises, sorted by Exercise Reference Number, as shown in Appendix F. Additional exercises are there too and you can choose an alternative from there if you prefer. The first letter denotes the body part targeted (Arms, Back, Chest,

Deltoids and Legs) – Deltoids are shoulders – and the next character denotes the type of exercise.

Chest: Press	C21 Seated Machine	C24 Smith Machine	C23 Dumbbells
Chest: Fly	C41 Seated Machine	C42 Standing Cables	C43 Dumbbells
Back: Pulldown	B43 Seated Machine	B42 Cable Leanback	B41 Cable Vertical
Back: Row	B31 Seated Machine	B32 Low Cable Row	B33 Single Arm Dumbbell Row
Legs: Upper	L33 Seat-Move Press	L32 Sled Leg Press	L31 Cradle Leg Press
Legs: Lower (Calf)	L53 Rotary Machine	L61 Seated Machine	L52 Standing Dumbbell Raise
Shoulders: Front	D12 Seated Machine	D11 Forward-Grip Dumbbells	D13 Rotational-Grip Dumbbells
Shoulders: Side	D32 Seated Machine	D31 Leaning Cable Raise	D34 Standing Dumbbells
Arms: Triceps	A31 Seated Machine	A21 Short Bar Pushdown	A11 Cable Centre Parting
Arms: Biceps	A51 Seated Machine	A44 Concentration Curl	A46 Barbell Preacher

1. Select the ten exercises you want to do, one from each row in this table or an alternative from Appendix F.

2. The sequence of the exercises isn't vital, but the usual practice is to train the largest muscle groups first, then smaller ones, which is how I've listed them. The largest ones need the most energy from you and it's best to do these first. You can then probably perform a small muscle exercise at the end, whereas you may have difficulty with a large one.

3. For each of your 10 selected exercises, perform 2 sets of 10 reps, leaving a minute's gap between each set. So, a total of 20 reps per exercise is the target – that is 200 reps per workout in total. Obviously, you perform 10 on each side for one-sided exercises to make a set.

4. The resistance doesn't change mid-set, of course, but it does after the end of the first set. If you completed all reps of the first set and with good form you increase the weight for the second set by the smallest possible increment. If the set is proving too heavy to complete with good form, don't finish it but end that set and reduce the resistance for the second set.

5. Make a written note of the weight on the second set. I'm not a fan of devices in the weights area because they can be broken, lost, trodden on or are a mental diversion to your workout. Old school pen and paper is best. You should also note any settings (seat position, height etc.) that are relevant for that exercise to help next time.

6. On your next workout, when you are doing the same exercise again, the resistance you used for the second set

last time, becomes the first weight this time. And it goes up for the second set this time as before. Always assuming that you complete the sets with good form, of course. In this way, the resistance goes up over time. For example, first visit = first set resistance 10, next at 11. Second visit = 11 and 12. Third visit = 12 and 13.

7. I recommend you consume a protein shake (ideally whey protein mixed with water) after the exercise, ideally between 15 and 30 minutes afterwards. That's when your muscles potentially benefit most from the effects of the protein.

There's a lot of information in this section and it may seem a daunting task to get to grips with it. If you haven't been in the weights area of a gym before there are many new practices to see and undertake and new terminology to learn. But, as with other things I've mentioned, you will get used to it and all is likely to become very familiar after a few gym visits.

If you need a guideline as to timing, this workout should probably take around 40 minutes. But it can take longer and no one is timing you. Don't rush anything to make a particular duration for the workout. If it is taking less than 40 minutes, I'll guess that your lower slower isn't slow enough.

Finally, should you find yourself caught up in massive enthusiasm for the gym and want to develop your gym routine further (don't laugh; I did!) then take a look at the Fit Happens Workout Plan and ABC7 System, both described on my Personal Training page[26].

Core Training Session

This is a training session that can take place at home or in the gym. It doesn't demand the use any special equipment, but you may find it easier on the mats in the gym; there are also one or two machines that you could use to help if you prefer to undertake this session in a gym. It should take around 15 minutes to perform.

I'll start off by specifying the area we are working on. By the core I mean the mid-section of the body – the front, sides and rear around your middle. The muscles involved are the stability and support muscles which support the spine, help your posture in terms of standing straight and add stability to your everyday movement. If someone accidentally pushes you, it's stability from your core that helps to stop you from falling over.

The other main function of the core is acting as the main hinge in the body. When you sit and move your chest and knees closer together, that's your core muscles. The mid-section also contains two other hinges, in the other two directions. If you do a sideways lean, maybe reaching one hand down the outer side of a leg, that is a movement of the mid-section, as is the final dimension, when your upper body twists. Those last two assume that the lower part of the body (pelvis downwards) is rigid; if it moves, that's cheating and probably shows that work on the side muscles of the core would be a good idea.

The first of those hinge motions is one of the functions of the famous 'six-pack' of muscles at the front of your mid-section, typically a few inches above and below your navel. You already have those six-pack muscles but you probably cannot see them, as they may be hidden behind a layer of bodyfat, and I suspect the muscles themselves could be strengthened. Not many people aged over fifty admit to wanting a visible six-pack (to confirm: that's not many *admit* to it), but for all that do I give you my number-one six-pack exercise – which doesn't form part of this training session, by the way. That exercise is to push your chair away from the table, to walk away and not to eat what's on the table.

OK, that was a bit of a joke, but the key point is that the six-pack isn't made visible solely by exercises targeted at the area. By far the major part of making the area visible is removing the layer of bodyfat over it. Certainly, exercise can develop the muscles to improve their function and appearance, but to actually see that hard work is much more about removing the fat layer than the exercise. You may have heard the old saying that 'abs aren't made through exercise; they are made through diet'. That's not really true, in reality they are developed through exercise, but made visible through diet. We are going to work on the exercise part in this session, the fat layer is being targeted by just about every other chapter of the book.

Any good mid-section training session will include exercises for the three hinge motions plus stability. I have examples, sorted by reference number, on my selection of exercise videos[27]. All my exercises that are for the mid-section begin with M.

We are going to cover those with five exercises in total – three that involve moving, and then two that don't. But that doesn't mean the final two are easy!

1. Firstly, let's work on the upper part of the front abs. These do their work when you move your chest towards your knees. That's not moving the knees, it's moving the chest. Typically, this would be a sit-up or a crunch type exercise, choose any from my list that begin with M1.

   As you do these exercises, perform them slowly, especially lower slower as your back comes down towards the floor. Each repetition should take at least three seconds, perhaps up to five. Don't lower so far that the back reaches the floor, because if you do you will lose tension in the abs, which is what we are trying to maintain. Abs develop as a result of continuous time under tension.

If your legs are stretched out in front, avoid weighing your feet down or having someone hold them down. Try to do that through your own effort. Keeping those legs on the ground is one of the functions of the mid-section.

Try a single set of a few reps, building up over time eventually to a single set of 30.

2. An exercise for the lower abs is next, that's the area south of the belly-button. For this area, pull the knees and pelvis up towards the chest. Typically, these would be leg raise or knee-up type exercises, and some examples begin M2 on my exercise videos.

   Again a slow pace is good, maintaining that continuous time under tension. Try to keep a slight hinge in place. If your legs are totally in line with your torso (such as when standing vertically), then the abs aren't involved and tension is lost. Continuous time under tension is important here too.

   As with the upper abs exercises, try a single set of a few reps building up over time eventually to a single set of 30.

3. The side muscles, or obliques, are the muscles that control twisting and leaning. The idea here is not to move the half of the body that isn't meant to move, such as in a sideways lean or an upper torso twist. Some examples are in my M3 series of exercises.

   It is good practice to alternate twist and lean motions on

different occasions of performing this training session. If you do a twist motion (such as a broomstick twist, M37) on one day, then next time on a core session you may want to tackle a leaning one, such as side bends (M32).

I recommend building up to a maximum of 20 repetitions on one side, then the same on the other.

4. It's now time to move to the stability functions and the two final exercises are planks or variations thereof.

The usual stationary plank is exercise M41, where you lie face-down on the floor up on your elbows, so that the points of contact with the ground are your toes and forearms. Keep the back straight, no camelbacks or U-bends in your plank please, and pull the tummy in as if someone's about to punch you there. Keep breathing at a normal pace, which can be a bit of an art while holding that position, but you will get used to it.

If you want some variations, including some with movement, any M4 exercise is fine. Ideally build up to 2 minutes for a stationary exercise or 20 reps of a moving one.

5. Finally, let's look at stability involvement for the obliques. At its simplest, start as a plank and rotate through 90 degrees so you are up on your side, the points of contact with the ground being one forearm and the side of one foot (the other foot rests on the first).

If you want to add some movement, try a side leg raise. Any M5 exercise is an example. Build up to 1 minute each side for a stationary exercise or 10 reps of a moving one.

Finally, if you attend an abs class at your gym, then that counts as this activity for that day.

Stretching Training Session

Again, this can take place at home or in the gym. There's no gym-only equipment needed, and it should take less time than the core training session – about 10 minutes.

This is an area where we are very much looking at the fitness-up aspect; there isn't much fat loss associated with stretching, although of course it will burn a few calories and will contribute towards your NEAT movement.

Flexibility is the ability to make a movement through its intended range of maximum motion without any restriction or pain. It is something that gradually gets lost over the years and, by the time someone is fifty, it is likely that they would not be able to move in the same range of motion as they could when younger. Stretching is the key to reversing that process.

As well as that impaired range of motion, a reduced ability to balance is often an effect of increased age, and this can be combatted in the same training session. There is also a concept called proprioception – that's the sense of where your body and its parts are at any time, which is linked to coordination. You may not want to be a master juggler, but you don't want to lose your ability to sense where limbs are and to move in a co-ordinated way. I call it the opposite of clumsy. Stretching and increased flexibility can help in this area too.

There are literally hundreds of different stretches possible, I have highlighted the ones that are the most beneficial for most people in a limited time. You can do your research if you want to look for more, or see a physiotherapist or specialist rehab therapist who can examine you and determine what stretches are ideal for you.

Here is a start-up set of stretches that seem to benefit most people. You can see photos of these stretches on my site.[28]

Each stretch is a static hold stretch (no bouncing) and takes 40 seconds if working both sides of the body. Many stretches are unilateral with 20 seconds each side. Note that the time given for each stretch is the time you should be in the full static stretching position, so you don't start your timing until you are in the fully stretched position and you don't relax from that position until the time is complete.

Start off by warming up by running on the spot for 30 seconds (high knees, please) or the same length of time in star jumps.

1. Calf

   Stand with toes of one foot touching the wall, that knee bent and also touching the wall, other foot far behind and also pointing forwards, hands and forehead on or very close to the wall. If you don't feel a great stretch in the rear calf, then straighten that leg by pressing the heel into the ground: 2 x 20 seconds.

2. Hamstrings

   Stand with one leg straight out in front, heel resting on a bench and foot pointing upwards. Bend forwards, reaching the arm and hand from the same side towards or to the toes, keeping the leg perfectly straight. Curling the toes towards you adds to the stretch: 2 x 20 seconds.

3. Quadriceps

   Kneel on the floor with buttocks on heels and knees slightly apart. Lean backwards. Leaning further backwards will increase the stretch. Lean the head slightly back, and arms can be crossed in front of the body or can be placed behind the back to add to the rearward and downward force: 40 seconds.

4. Rear aspect of shoulders

Stand upright and pull one arm straight and horizontally across the chest. Push that arm into place towards the shoulder by the thumb edge of the other hand, which should be pressing at the elbow. The elbow of the side being stretched can be bent or straight: 2 x 20 seconds.

5. Triceps

Stand and move one arm to a vertical position upwards, then reach over and behind at the elbow so your fingers reach to the shoulder blade, the elbow being pushed backwards by the thumb edge of the other hand and alongside the ear. Use your fingertips to gradually walk down the backbone to increase the stretch: 2 x 20 seconds.

6. Chest

Stand in a doorframe alongside the non-hinge side as if you were walking through the doorway leaving a room. Keep your side forearm and part of the upper arm against the wall inside the room. Keep the forearm vertical and the elbow bent at 90 degrees. Walk a little way forward, stabilising yourself with a split stance. The further forward you stand, the greater the stretch: 2 x 20 seconds.

7. Shoulders

Lie flat on the floor, face-up, arms alongside ears so that the hands are as far from the feet as possible. The palms should be upwards and knuckles on the floor. Stretch further to straighten the arms – the heels, buttocks, shoulder blades, back of the head, elbows and knuckles should all touch the floor. Use a dumbbell or another object to reach towards, if that helps: 40 seconds.

Finally, this is not really a stretch but a good proprioceptive way to end. Stand on one leg for 40 seconds, then the same on the other.

If you attend a yoga class that includes stretching, then that counts as this activity for that day.

Conclusion

If you achieve performing a core, stretching or weight training session on a day, then enter a 1 for that day under the Train column when you have your Daily Data spreadsheet open. If you didn't achieve that, you should enter a 0.

You can use the vacant column to the right to make a note of which of the three types of training you performed that day, Core, Stretching or Weights, if that helps keep a track of the 2+2+3 breakdown. I have done this in the sample format of the Daily Data Sheet, Appendix G.

18 – Your Daily Data Spreadsheet

We've now looked at all ten of the daily objectives. If you haven't already started to do so, this is where you record your achievements on the Daily Data sheet and track your progress. You will be using your Daily Data sheet for this together with figures from MyFitnessPal and your activity tracker.

Setting up the sheet was described in Chapter 8 and you can find a suggested format for this in Appendix G. There are just a couple of further pieces of advice on formatting as we start to enter data.

The Weight-Average and Bodyfat-Average columns are designed to be used as a seven-day moving average of the values in the columns immediately to their left respectively. These average columns are a more reliable indicator of your performance as they even out any day-to-day variances arising from one-off conditions. Sometimes these can be as simple as how recently you've been to the loo, when you last drank any water, if you've had a particularly excessive day on eating or drinking, or things you only do on certain days of the week such as at weekends. They can all make the day's figures show an atypical reading and be dispiriting, so I always suggest using those seven-day moving averages as your guide to progress.

Set the seven-day moving averages for any day by defining the contents of that cell to be the sum of the cell to its left, plus the six cells above, all divided by seven. Obviously, that only works after you have recorded seven days of data. Up to that point, you have to base your average on a smaller number of days.

You may wish to total the ten objective-achieved columns and also sum across the totals. This way you can see which areas are performing better than others. This has been done in Appendix G, where you can see the user achieved 40 out of the 70 objectives.

When do you enter the data? You may assume that the best time to do this is at the end of each day. With experience, I have found that this is not the case. First thing in the morning is the best time to record that day's data from the scales, and the previous day's performance on the ten objectives, and update MyFitnessPal. Why is morning better? Several reasons:

1. You definitely have finished yesterday's activities by the next morning, so you won't miss anything. For example, the calories burned between going to bed and midnight will be included.

2. People are often tired at night and the last thing you want to be doing is opening spreadsheets late and getting the brain wound up, as that won't help you sleep well. Screen time before bed is not conducive to good sleep in any case.

3. You are going to open the Daily Data sheet tomorrow morning anyway to enter that day's weight and bodyfat percentage, so you can enter yesterday's performance data on the objectives at the same time. This way you only need to open the sheet once per day.

4. Yesterday's results from both MyFitnessPal and the Daily Data sheet will be fresh in your mind if you see them in the morning of the new day. That way it's much better then to plan for the coming day, making any adjustments to your plans for that day that seem a good idea bearing in mind the results from yesterday.

That does have the consequence of making the morning task list look quite lengthy. But once you've done it a few times you will find it takes less than a couple of minutes. That time is well worth the amount of useful information you can derive from it, believe me.

Here is a summary of the suggested morning activity:

1. On the scales, make a note of that day's weight and bodyfat.

2. Create a new row in your Daily Data spreadsheet for today's date by copying the row above and pasting below. You can see where we are heading with this in the sample format shown in Appendix G.

3. Overtype the values for weight and bodyfat that have been copied down with today's values. Check that the moving averages are working. Blank out all the 0 and 1 values that are yesterday's and have been copied down.

4. On MyFitnessPal – close yesterday by selecting the Complete Diary function at the top then review yesterday's nutrition (turning the phone on its side to a landscape view if that works better). Note the results that MyFitnessPal tells you about yesterday's calories consumed, and grams of protein, sugar, fat and saturated fat consumed.

5. If you have a smartwatch or phone-based activity tracker, use it to see calories burned yesterday, perform a subtraction from the MyFitnessPal number for calories consumed to give a calorie deficit for yesterday (hopefully not a surplus too often). If you don't have an activity tracker, do the same using your TOC number compared to yesterday's calories consumed on MyFitnessPal. You are determining if you achieved your calorie deficit target for yesterday.

6. Enter a 1 or 0 in the relevant columns of the first five of the yes/no columns (the five linked to what you consumed yesterday) that's a 1 if you achieved your target, or a 0 if you didn't.

7. Enter a 1 or 0 in the relevant columns for the other objectives – Ate and drank only in the planned twelve hours? Performed a single, continuous 30-minute cardio session during the day? Did you drink a significant amount of water that day? Did your step-counter show you achieved your target daily steps? And finally, did you undertake a period of training yesterday, being one of the weights, core, or stretching sessions?

8. You may want to enter which of those three training sessions you performed on an additional column to the right of 'Train', to help ensure you have an even spread of types of session over the week.

9. Take a minute or two to look at the data. This isn't an input-only system, and this is an 'informal' review'; you won't be resetting targets from it, but maybe you may want to change some aspects of what you do today based on what you see. Remember to use the moving average values for weight and bodyfat.

10. Finally, while you have MyFitnessPal to hand, now would be a great time to enter today's plan for eating in the MyFitnessPal Diary bearing in mind what was good, and not so good, yesterday. Enter items for the full day ahead even though you haven't started eating yet.

When you've done all that, put on some sports clothing, grab a black tea or coffee and go for your morning cardio.

All this work in MyFitnessPal and the Daily Data sheet may sound onerous. I guarantee it won't be when (a) you see the weight and bodyfat percentage numbers move in the right direction, and (b) you get used to it. It will all be an input to your weekly review, and that's coming in Chapter 20.

If you don't like the thought of all this data, remember those who keep daily records typically lose twice as much weight as those that don't. That's an extension of my saying about what gets written, gets done.

Finally, a bit more repetition. No apologies because this is important and I want to make sure the message hits home. I'm not asking you to follow 100% my suggestions for 100% of the time. That just isn't going to work. You'll make a success of it by following most of my suggestions most of the time. The higher the percentages are, the sooner the desired outcome is likely to be achieved. But high levels of adherence are not possible in the real world. You have a life outside of your lifestyle upgrade programme. Live your real life, but always keep an eye on the fitness aspects of what you are doing. Initially you will have to remember to do that but soon it will become second nature.

19 – A Sample Day

There have been some substantial portions of guidance over the past chapters. Here I bring all those individual, discrete pieces of advice and recommendations together into an example day, with real foods to consider. I hope this helps you see how you can successfully make all the aspects of the plan work for you.

Of course, I know nothing of your work, family, medical or other commitments. It's for you to overlay those into this sample schedule.

For food and drink, I list five numbers after each item on this sample schedule. These are numbers of calories, then grams of protein, sugar, fats and saturated fats in each item. Numbers are rounded and are based on figures on nutrition labels and in MyFitnessPal. Often these don't add up totally accurately but they are close.

I have chosen 2000 calories as the TIC (Target Inwards Calories) with at least 150g of protein and maximums of 67g of sugar and 67g of fats including 20g of saturates. These are the relevant figures based on a 2000-calorie day from Chapter 11.

This is reproduced from my nutrition on an actual day that I was outside my Target Zone. I used the same day as an example of my own nutrition in Part One of the book. It is a day when eating is at five times: breakfast, lunch, afternoon (part one), afternoon (part two) and evening. The approach I have used is approximately 500 calories for each part of the day, splitting the afternoon in two.

The nutrition numbers are reproduced in table form in Appendix J.

The first thing is to weigh yourself, taking a note of the weight and bodyfat percentage. Either now or later during the morning, update the Daily Data Sheet with yesterday's results and add today's planned eating into MyFitnessPal.

- The first item consumed is a black coffee. Zero calories, to provide caffeine as a stimulant and help promote bodyfat burning as fuel. No calories, so it doesn't count as a meal.

- Then it's off to the gym for the HIT or MISS cardio, then shower and home. Keep well-hydrated during and immediately after the cardio, probably around a litre of water in total if you've been sweating, mainly afterwards.

- 9am is a good time for breakfast, which could be a Power Breakfast. This is based on oats with hot water with berries and nuts. I describe it in detail in Appendix D. It includes a half a litre of whey protein shake with a single scoop of protein powder made with water. *(540/32/10/21/4)*

- 12 noon is perhaps time for meal two, lunch. As an example, it could be spaghetti carbonara with mixed vegetables on the side, followed by a low-calorie yoghurt and water. *(453/30/20/6/3)*

- Maybe go for training at 2pm, which could be weights. Drink another 0.5 litre of water. On leaving the gym, increase the protein with 50g of low-carb whey protein shake and an apple, which is the first half of meal three. The protein is less important if this is a stretching or abs training session. *(252/38/11/4/2)*

- Part two of the afternoon calories is maybe at 4pm. This could be a high-protein, low-sugar snack bar if you happened to have a sweet tooth. Many manufacturers and flavours are available, the example here are the numbers for Grenade 'Carb Killa' Bar in Dark Chocolate Mint flavour. *(214/22/1/9/5)*

- The final meal can perhaps be at 7pm. A suggestion is beef and ale stew with some small amounts of bacon and more mixed veg, followed by a treat of a calorie-controlled chocolate mousse. *(537/69/25/12/5)*

- This is a good time to check your step count for the day, and go for a brisk walk if you need to increase it to reach your target.

- Keep the water up throughout the day, 1 litre as part of the two protein shakes and another 1.5 accompanying cardio and training workouts, plus whatever further water you feel like. That ensures that 2.5 litres are taken. You can have black tea and coffee during the day and maybe one (maximum) zero calorie soda, drinks with no calories and no macronutrients.

The spread of calories is 9am to 7pm, just 10 hours – you could spread things out further and still maintain the 12-hour overnight fast.

That adds up to 1996 calories, 192 grams of protein, 67 grams of sugar and 51 grams of fats of which 18 grams are saturates. These numbers are within the target of 2000/200/67/67/20. Much of this calculation and measuring is estimation of course, not only by me also by the manufacturers, so it is not as accurate as those total numbers suggest.

That sample day would probably achieve a full spread of 1 values in the final columns of your Daily Data sheet. As I've said multiple times, you don't need to do that always to be successful on the plan.

20 – The Weekly Stage Two Review

One thing you will be definitely be looking forward to is reviewing your progress at intervals. A week is the perfect length of time between reviews and you can plan to look at the data ideally on the same day each week. This is when you check the results revealed by your Daily Diary sheet and make some decisions about what you see.

The first thing to check is: are you in your Target Zone now? We defined that back in Chapter 5 and it is the state you are in when both your weight and bodyfat are at or better than the targets you set for them. If the latest average readings say that you are, then its big congratulations to you! You should now head on to Stage Three in the next chapter. Of course, it's unlikely that you're in the Target Zone in the early stages of following the plan – especially if the target date that you set is still some way ahead.

If you are not in the Target Zone now, then this means you need to continue with Stage Two. I suggest you make the border under the last day on the Daily Data sheet into a thicker line (format cells, border is the function in Excel). That really does draw a line under the previous week and sets you up for a new week.

Now see if you are moving in the right direction. Check today's average numbers for weight and bodyfat, and compare them with the equivalent numbers from this time last week (or compare with the starting values if this is your first weekly review). Are they heading in the right direction, towards your Target Zone?

What you do next:

1. If both the numbers are moving in the right direction, then you are well on track to reaching your target values. This is exactly what we want and you are doing great! I wouldn't advise changing anything at this point. Continue as you are and see if you're still making progress this time next week.

2. Your weight has gone down but not the bodyfat percentage is one possibility. It is good news that you are losing bodyfat, but not that you are losing muscle mass. In most cases this suggests that you have reduced the quantity of food, but that the quality isn't quite where it should be. Review the 1 and 0 values from the week just ended. Add extra emphasis on keeping the protein up, sugars and fats down, and keeping within your Target Input Calories number. Water is important to help muscles thrive, so try adding extra hydration through the course of the day. You could increase the weight training to a definite three times per week (on non-adjacent days), making sure that you are progressing incrementally to heavier resistances.

3. You bodyfat percentage has gone down but not your weight. This is a very rare outcome. It suggests you have lost bodyfat and added the same amount of muscle/water – not the worst outcome by a long way. But you may be drinking too much water. Try another week to see if the result differs.

4. Your weight and bodyfat percentage have both gone up, which not what we wanted. It suggests you need to 'turn up the dial' on the ten objectives. Review the 1 and 0 values from the week just ending and see if there is a pattern. Are there particular columns which reveal a lower level of achievement of specific objectives? If so try to find ways to increase that level of adherence to the objectives for next week. If you have a good spread of 1 values from the week ending, then one tactic is to

reset the nutrition numbers, maybe changing your Target Input Calories down by 100, and making the appropriate adjustments to other nutrition variables, using the table or percentages in Chapter 11 to guide you. Adding to your daily step count is another way of helping here.

If you find your weight and bodyfat continue to increase after a second week with a high level of achievement of the ten objectives, then a discussion with a professional dietician would be useful. Probably stop by your GP first and explain why this is being suggested to you.

As I said much earlier, there's nothing in the chapters before this that I haven't tried myself, and I only recommend actions to you because they were successful when I did them. I believe that the majority of my recommendations will prove similarly successful for the majority of readers. However, I know that everybody is different, so I can't guarantee that everything that worked for me in my fat-down, fit-up journey will have worked for you.

If it hasn't worked, feel free to send me an email describing your activity and results and I will give further thought to your unique situation and see if I can suggest alternative approaches. If you do visit a dietician as I mentioned above, I would be keen to hear what is suggested.

21 – All Good Things

I bet you were wondering if Stage 3 would ever make an appearance. Well, here it is – the final chapter.

Stage 3 means you are in your Target Zone. Life is moving from good to better. If you want to, you can put all the fitness activities away and file this book in the deepest recesses of your bookshelf or hard drive. You've achieved what you set out to achieve.

However, if you're anything like me (and now that you have read tens of thousands of my words, I feel we are converging at some level) then you will want to continue your life maintaining your own fitness as a high priority. It would be a waste to go from where you are now to being inactive and eating too many of the wrong kind of calories. I would wager that your tastes have moved on and that you no longer crave foots high in sugar and fat.

On the movement side I am going to make another prediction: that is, I suspect that you have had your own Magic Moment by now and that you are enjoying some or all of the exercise you are undertaking. If I said you couldn't do any more running, or other cardio, or brisk walking, or weight training, core work or stretching, my money is on the fact that you would regret that. You are doing it now because you actually enjoy it, not because you are doing so for health reasons.

If you need any suggestions as to how to live your lifestyle in this fitness-maintenance mode, take a look back at the twelve guidelines of Stage One in Chapter 6. Adopt any or all of those to the extent that you feel comfortable.

One thing you probably should keep an eye on, especially as you still have the body composition monitor in the bathroom, is your bodyfat and weight. Having achieved your Target Zone, you don't want to let go so much that you slip outside it. But if you do, you know what to do: go back to the guidelines of Stage One, and if that doesn't sort it, it is Stage Two for you.

You know me well by now and are probably fed up with my quotes and sayings. A couple of people who are not have asked me to include a summary of them, so it's the last thing in the book, Appendix Z. There's nothing there you haven't seen before if you've read the whole book. Some may make you smile though, especially with hindsight. And if you have any favourite fitness sayings that you have invented, feel free to email them to me and I may update Appendix Z with them for the next edition.

Before we say goodbye, a couple of requests from me.

If you enjoy running as your cardio and you decide to take up parkrun, do let me know and also the location of your home parkrun. Jenny and I visit parkrun locations around the UK (and sometimes beyond) and it would be good to share a coffee afterwards with you.

Finally, if this book has helped you, please document your own fat-to-fit-at-fifty success story. Email it to me and I'll include it on my website, blog or monthly newsletter. Perhaps include a photo or two if you are willing to share them, maybe before and after images. You've done something really special and I want to help you to share it.

It has added years to your life, and life to your years.

Thanks

There are many people I want to thank for their support in my life, for help in writing the book, or both. Each person has played his or her own part in my story and making this a book I believe worth writing by me, and I hope worth reading by you.

Firstly, I thank my wonderful wife Jenny who has helped me every step of the way. She has always been there when I needed some unrestricted kisses to go with the restricted calories, and continues to champion my fitness journey to this day, despite her injury. We look forward to a time in a few years when that will no longer be a factor in our lives.

I am grateful to everybody I've mentioned in the text. They have all helped me in their own ways, and I remain friends with them all. In particular I thank Rob Riches in California for his inspiration, motivation and education, all of which I needed especially in my early days in the gym. And Dan Wynes, who initially asked me to guide him, and ended up guiding me.

I'm very lucky to have several workout buddies that regularly share workouts with me. They all realise that a workout shared is social time and exercise time bundled together, while helping each other progress, all in an hour or less. In particular (from north to south in the UK) – Rob, Nicola, Mark, Lorna, David, Oggie, Fraser, Blue, Neil, Manoj, Graeme and Andy.

Of course, I want to express my thanks to all my personal training clients past and present, all of whom turned my fitness activity into my business activity. In this group, I am especially grateful to Nick Bowers who was kind enough to write his own thoughts as an appendix.

Thanks too to the professional photographers who have allowed their images to appear here – Simon Howard and Matt Marsh. Professionals both, and friends, too.

I am very keen to acknowledge the generous time of Chris, George, Jenny, Roger and Shawn for proof-reading this book and spotting so many errors. All those that remain are mine.

Finally, I thank you for reading my book. If you have followed the guidance, and have made your own fat-down, fit-up transformation, please let me know as I mentioned at the end of the last chapter. I can then thank you personally.

Appendix A – Nick's Story

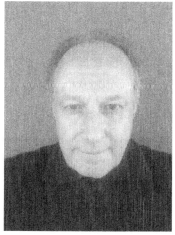

It's another lovely morning. I have awoken with a clear plan ahead for a productive day. I will follow the methods and wise counsel of Chris Zaremba and keep fitter, leaner and more focused.

Before I met Chris, I knew I was overweight and not in good shape. I was in my mid-fifties and had worked in the City for thirty years. As a younger man I was, as they say, naturally fit.

I played sport, ran two London marathons and I burned calories with ease. As I became older things changed. My body stored my poor diet as fat, muscles began to diminish and weaken. I knew something had to be done.

I had used personal trainers before, but this time I wanted someone of my own generation to be my coach. After much online research I found 'Fitness over Fifty'. Damascus was signposted. I was on the road to having a weight off my body and my mind.

Other than me being an overweight, unfit office worker and Chris being a world champion and personal trainer, we had much in common. Chris had also worked in the City and decided to change his physical condition and life. We shared an optimistic outlook, a love of ancient popular music and a penchant for terrible jokes. Gym sessions were to be full of laughter and song as well as focused hard work.

Our first session was an assessment of my physical condition. The word 'obese' was never said but the statistics never lie. Having accepted and confronted the challenge, progress commenced.

In essence improving your fitness and losing weight is very simple. Through eating healthy food, exercise and resistance training you burn more calories than you consume and you build muscle. If you follow such a programme the statistics will record your progress and success with clinical precision. In many aspects of life, you need the help of others or good fortune to be successful. Not so in respect of fitness. It is rooted in science. If you take the right approach and apply it consistently nothing will stop you succeeding. It is up to you.

Chris's programme is, as mentioned, made of three core elements – cardio, resistance (weight) training and good nutrition. Chris would oversee two weight training sessions per week and the cardio and nutrition programme was up to me to follow. I was measured on electronic scales every session for my weight and for muscle and fat percentages. Targets were set for specific time periods. As there was a remarkable correlation between adherence to the plan and improving statistics it was very motivating.

For me one of the keys to success was maintaining a daily food diary and I would recommend this approach. I sent Chris a record of each day's consumption and cardio and he would make constructive comments. I used email but of course there is sophisticated technology for recording and measuring on your phone or on a watch. Multiple incentives are at play. The desire to score well, personal pride, the wish to impress your coach, the clarity of having the data for self-analysis and the satisfaction of consistent progression. Another benefit of a diary is that if you go off track a couple days of good work can return you to the right path.

So, what might a perfect Zaremba diary day look like?

7 00 Espresso Coffee

7 15 5k run or cycling for an hour

8 00 Porridge with whey protein and blueberries

10 30 4 Turkey slices

13 00 Smoked salmon with avocado

16 00 4 more Turkey slices or a protein bar

17 00 Resistance training with Chris

18 30 Chicken or fish with roast vegetables. Glass of red wine....

I was working in an office during this typical day and the weight training recorded was twice a week. I think Chris would give the diary entry pretty good marks.

Let's examine some of Chris's simple principles which lie behind the day – many of which are in this book.

7 00 – After you wake up is a great time to burn fat. The body has been burning calories throughout the night and further exercise will stimulate the body to burn fat as fuel. Don't add calories but a coffee to get the heart pumping. Now let's run, cycle, cross training or walk fast to keep the cardio burning fat.

8 00 – A slow burning natural carb like oats combined with a protein like whey respectively provides slow burn energy and builds muscle for the day. Wonderful. Building muscle is marvellous as it in turn uses energy and calories.

10 30 – Eat often and in small quantities. A mid-morning protein snack staves off any unwanted hunger pangs and helps that muscle build. Eating something healthy also reduces the risk of eating something unhealthy through boredom.

13 00 – Lunch. A combination of protein and healthy carbs. Note the absence of man-made (processed) carbs during the course of day. You know that bread, biscuits, cake and so on are unhealthy. Yes, it is the science of sugars and starches quickly turning to fat, but it is also good old fashioned common sense!

16 00 – An afternoon protein snack will take you through to the end of any day when you might be flagging. Yes, a protein bar is man-made but the right ones are low in sugar and high in protein. So much better than a biscuit or chocolate bar!

17 00 – A weight/resistance session with Chris. Time to measure progress since the last meeting then a focus on specific muscle groups. Achieve personal bests for extra motivation. Everything is recorded. Many bad jokes are told and vintage hits are hummed to. Marvellous.

18 30 – More protein builds the muscles after weight training and the vegetables provide healthy carbohydrates. The glass of red wine has some health benefits and is less calorific than white but in truth it is a weakness.

I stuck to a programme similar to this for six months, lost three stones, built a better physique and felt tremendous. It was a great fun. We all have different nutritional likes and dislikes-many are vegans or vegetarians-but the core Zaremba principles apply.

Chris has been an inspiration and I have signed up to become a fitness instructor – it's down to him. When things get tough out running or in the gym, I say two magic words... 'Remember Zaremba'. Just the sort of awful, lame joke we might laugh about in the gym.

Thanks for everything Chris. You took a weight off my body and my mind.

Nick Bowers

Appendix B – Cardio Training

This appendix both describes what I do for cardio training, and what I recommend for others generically. It may not work perfectly for everyone, and of course the standard health advisories apply. If you can't run, then perhaps double the MISS and give the HIT a miss, so to speak.

MISS Training

This is a 40-minute session on the cross-trainer which typically burns around 400 to 500 calories according to the display. Keep moving in time to the music of headphones or the gym's own speakers, and adjusting the resistance level to keep the heart rate in the target range for as much of the duration as possible.

Of course, it's difficult to keep exactly at one specific heart rate, so an acceptable range is a heart rate which is 75% (Medium Intensity) of the maximum heart rate plus or minus 2. So, at age 55 the maximum heart rate is 165 (from the calculation earlier, 220 minus age). In this example, 75% is 124, therefore the acceptable range is 122-126. If the heart rate is within that, all is fine, change nothing. Below that, move the resistance up by one; above and of course it's down by one.

To save constantly changing the resistance levels, check only on the minute and change by one increment at that time. It usually takes 5-10 minutes to get a heart rate up to those levels, but once it's there, do those on-the-minute adjustments to keep it there.

I sometimes use the handles on the machine, sometimes not, and typically do alternating periods of 5 minutes of each. Use of the handles involves the upper body in a bit of workout, is a little more efficient at calorie burning (as there are more body parts in action), whereas using just the legs to power the cross-trainer leaves my hands free. When I'm legs-only, I do stuff on my phone – including planning the day ahead and handling emails. I don't like phones in the weights area of gyms, but I'm fine with phones and cardio – if I'm listening or watching it, I'm unlikely to leave it behind or it heading to the floor.

If I am using handles, then I'm often watching the news (with subtitles so I keep my music) or maybe something else on the video screen that gives some level of interest. My current gym has internet connectivity for the screen on each cross-trainer, so I can check out a few YouTube videos if I want. All to keep the brain occupied while those bodyfat-sourced calories are being used up. I recommend you try those approaches.

HIT Training

The pattern I use for my 30-miute HIT sessions is complicated, but works well for me. The calories burned indication will typically be in the range of 250-300, but all the treadmills I know do not include the excess calorie burn during slowdown, the real benefit of HIT.

Start the HIT sessions at a certain speed that is known to be comfortable – say at a speed of 6mph (9kph), which is a standard setting on many treadmills – then run for 2 minutes at that speed. Then slow right down to a slow walking pace, say 2mph (3kph); again, that is often a standard setting.

Keep walking at that speed until the heart rate is back to a low intensity number – at example age 55, I would use 107, which is

65% (Low Intensity) of the theoretical maximum. Since you aren't running for that time you can use the heart rate monitor on the machine (if fitted) if you don't have your own. I wouldn't advise using that while running, it disrupts the normal flow of the running movement, but it's fine during the slow walking intervals.

Once the heart rate has reached that target number, switch up and go fast again for the next two-minute period. Then slow walk again back down to 107, or whatever is your low figure. This cycling up-down pattern continues until the 30 minutes is completed.

I find it interesting to see how each walking period turns out to be longer than the preceding one, as it is taking longer to get back to that Low Intensity figure; obviously the heart rate recovery slows down as the number of intervals increase during the 30 minutes.

I add a few complexities in. I wouldn't be myself if I kept it too simple, especially with loads of numbers around to play with.

Firstly, the initial two-minute fast run is actually not two minutes – there is a warm-up element. So that first two-minute high-speed session actually comprises one minute at half the target speed, then the second minute at the selected speed. I do this an introduction into the run, and its only on the very first interval each time I do the exercise.

Secondly, I nudge the speed up for each fast interval by the smallest increment available on the treadmill. So, if my first two minutes was at 6mph (ignoring the warm-up modification) then my second two-minute fast – after the first slow walk – will be at 6.1mph, and the third at 6.2mph and so on. This gradual increment also contributes to the longer recovery time required in the walking periods for the heart rate to get back to that low figure. These slow periods are always at 2mph.

A third complexity is that I try to have the starting speed itself increasing over time. I link this progression to my increase in fitness, which I measure by a reduction in walking time, which itself I measure by the number of completed high-speed intervals I complete in the previous HIT session. I keep track of the number of 2-minute runs I perform and if I find I have completed eight or more high-speed intervals, then I'll shift the initial high-speed value next time up by 0.1mph.

As an example, I started with a run at 6mph (again, ignoring the warm-up modification), then if I have fully completed eight running segments – the final one will have been two minutes at 6.7mph – then I'll start my next session with an initial high-speed value of 6.1mph (modified by warm-up). This enables me to progress over time based on my fitness level, measuring that fitness by time taken for heart rate recovery – one of the indicators of increasing fitness.

I suggest you consider adopting all three of these enhancements to the basic approach. It enables you to show progress, and keeps it interesting while slightly increasing calorie burn rate as the months pass. It may all seem complicated at this stage, but stick with it and follow the guidelines; soon it will be second nature.

These days I keep all the data for my HIT sessions on a phone-based spreadsheet app, so I can easily compare numbers such as initial speed, completed high-speed segments, distance run, maximum heart rate and calories burnt and see how they progress over time. I also have the data ready for next time, such as knowing what my first high-speed should be based on my number of completed segments. Again, I recommend that for you – although a notepad will work just as well.

Appendix C – Healthy Food Choices

Here are some of the good, the less good, and the ugly items on the food front. These are high-level guidelines for you to use until (or if) you are on Stage Two of the Fat to Fit at Fifty plan. At that point, you will be guided more by the ingredients, nutrients and calorie content rather than a simple description such as this list.

The list doesn't cover everything, and some of the items really deserve a kind of further intermediate category, but it should point you in the right direction when you are in the supermarket (which is towards the first list) and in the fried fast-food joint (which is towards the exit).

Eat lots (including protein, good carbs):

- Meats (trim excess fat and skin)
- Fish
- Shellfish
- Eggs
- Protein shakes
- Slow-absorbing carbs with fibre such as green stuff, leafy veg, tomatoes, salad
- Items both low in carbs and fat, such as Fage Zero Greek yoghurt
- Products with all green traffic light labelling
- Coffee / tea
- Water

Eat some:

- Fresh fruit (an acceptable fast carb)
- Oily fish (tuna, mackerel, salmon, trout, sardines)
- Meat with fat that can't be cut off (marbled steak)
- Low fat dairy including fully skimmed milk
- Wholemeal (brown) rice
- Potatoes – but only baked, including the skin
- Beans
- Good bread (wholemeal)
- Nuts and seeds
- Diet drinks
- Products with amber traffic light labelling
- Starchy / root veg (carrots, swedes, sweet potatoes)
- Great quality beer and wine (to be social)
- Oils for cooking – look for extra virgin olive oil or any mentioning Omega-3

Eat rarely (mainly sugars or low-quality fats):

- Sausages, bacon and other processed meats
- Dried or canned fruit
- Breakfast cereals with any form of sugar
- White stuff (rice, bread, pasta, crackers, croutons)
- Chips, fried potatoes and processed potato products
- Fatty sauces
- Cakes, pastries, biscuits, sweets, chocs, desserts
- Full fat milk, yoghurts and other dairy
- Butter and similar, honey and jam
- Fruit juice, coke and other soft/fizzy drinks (non-diet)
- Low quality beer and wine
- Products with a red traffic light labelling
- Anything else with salt or high levels of sugar
- Anything with a large proportion of saturated fats, or any trans fats

Three additional principles:

> Look for natural, whole, unprocessed items – minimise
> processed and refined.

> Generally, grilled, baked or microwaved is best, avoid fried,
> especially deep-fat fried.

> The fewer ingredients something has, usually the better it is for
> you.

Appendix D – Power Breakfast

It's often said that breakfast is the most important meal of the day. There are some great breakfast ways to start the day, plus a few lousy ones – I considered including the phrase 'Cereal Killers' at this point.

My favourite breakfast is the Power Breakfast that we have enjoyed in our house every day for over ten years, after having been awake for a couple of hours and completed my morning cardio. This has helped me to both build muscle and lose fat, and I can't see me changing it anytime soon. Here are the details:

There are four key principles behind the breakfast:

- Portion size – big enough to provide sufficient amounts of nutrients both long-term for the day ahead and shorter-term for the next three to four hours before the next meal.

- Macronutrient ratio – compared to most people's breakfasts, the Power Breakfast has a higher protein amount and lower carb content, and the fats come from natural sources and are unsaturated.

- Minimise sugar – we need some carbs but not the many of the fast-absorbing ones that can potentially cause blood sugar to spike. Some fast carbs from a natural source would be helpful to start the day.

- Quality ingredients – everything as natural as possible with the minimum of processing involved in getting it to the table.

The first step is to add a small amount of very hot (not boiling) water to a bowl containing 65g of rolled oats. That may be more oats than you're used to, and with less water than you'd expect, as more liquid is coming later. These are simple, basic rolled oats, with nothing added by the supplier. I prefer jumbo or steel-cut.

The oats are a medium-speed digested carbohydrate, and this amount provides 39g of carb with virtually no sugar – a key benefit of oats. There are small amounts of incomplete protein and fat here, but it's really the energy-giving slow-digesting carbs we're after from the oats.

While the oats are cooling, make a whey protein shake with 25g of product in around a half-litre of cold water. There are many suppliers of whey protein, and you may already have your favourite supplier and flavours. After years of experimentation, I always chose chocolate these days. The 25g serving is usually one scoop for most manufacturers, and provides 19g of quality protein. There are also small amounts of carbs and fats, but it's the protein that counts here.

Add a few nuts to the top of the oats. Keep it to around 25g in total – I used mixed nuts, available at supermarkets. Without fruit or salt or roasting – as natural as possible. There's around 13g of (mainly unsaturated) fats here, as well as small amounts of the other two macros.

Next to be added are a few berries – typically about 50g but, as with the nuts, I 'eyeball' the quantity rather than weighing daily. The berries are always of mixture of any two from blueberries, raspberries and blackberries. These berries are amongst the lowest on the glycaemic index of any fruits. And this is where the small amount of fast-acting carbs, the sugar, comes from – plus useful micronutrients including vitamins, minerals and antioxidants.

Then add some of the protein shake to the bowl and give it a stir. The amount depends on how liquid you like your oats, but for me it's usually about 10% of the prepared shake, the first inch or so from a glass. This is where the flavour of the shake is important, as it turns the taste of the oats into the flavour of the shake. This is why It's always a chocolate-based flavour that gets my vote; I like my oats chocolatey!

The remainder of the shake stays in the glass and is a drink to be consumed alongside the oats. This is needed for the full amount of protein in for the meal, and is a great alternative to sugar-heavy orange or other fruit juice as your breakfast drink.

The final element is a sprinkling of ground cinnamon over the top, a spice that acts as a thermogenic to raise the metabolism and help burn fat, and adds a slight contrasting taste on the tongue.

This meal (including the drink) provides around 540 calories, as shown below. It's around 24% of calories from protein, 39% from carbs (but only 7% from sugars) and 35% from fats (but under 7% from saturates). A perfect way to start the day for me and others who like more protein and less carbs than most breakfasts!

For the numbers fans, here's the rounded breakdown of the Power Breakfast, the oats and drink combined showing the grams of each nutrient. As is often the case, the numbers don't add up exactly the way they should – different manufacturers obviously use slightly different algorithms:

	Kcal	Protein	Sugar	Fats	Sat Fats	Carbs
Oats 65g	244	7	0	5	1	39
Shake 25g	100	19	1	2	1	2
Nuts 25g	154	5	1	13	1	2
Berries 50g	42	1	7	0	0	11
	540	32	10	21	4	53

Appendix E – Stage One Workout

Here's a workout I've designed for people at Stage One of the plan. The workout features strength exercises for all the major muscle groups, plus core strengthening and some flexibility movements.

You can see a video of the workout to see how each exercise is performed[29]. Here are some notes to go with the video:

1. Warm up, being 30 seconds of running on the spot then 30 seconds of jumping jacks.

2. Strength exercises: 10 repetitions of each as a single set - adding more repetitions and a second set when comfortable

    2.1 Chest - Press-ups (push-ups) perhaps easier kneeling variant

    2.2 Upper legs (1) - Air squats, keeping arms horizontal

    2.3 Back - Door pulls, ideally overhand grip

    2.4 Calf - Step raises, full range up and down

    2.5 Shoulders - Seated press, down to ear height

    2.6 Upper legs (2) - Raised lunges, 10 each side

    2.7 Biceps - Keeping upper arms welded to side torso

    2.8 Upper legs (3) - Bottle squats, keep head up + facing front.

3. Core exercises: for abs area as a stabilisation or fixator muscle group - again start from 10 repetitions (or 10 each side) and build up

> 3.1 Elbow plank - keeping body straight - try 30 seconds and build up to 2 minutes

> 3.2 Upper abs - curling the chest and upper body towards the knees, low and slow

> 3.3 Side abs or obliques - twist as far as possible each side

> 3.4 Lower abs - bringing the knees and lower body towards the chest.

4. Flexibility and balance - hold 20 seconds of each (or each side)

> 4.1 Quads - best done with backside touching heels

> 4.2 Hamstrings - keeping knees locked, curl toes towards head

> 4.3 Calf - ensure rear leg locked straight and heel flat on ground

> 4.4 Upper back and rear deltoid - stretch by maximising range

> 4.5 Triceps - walk the fingers down the vertebrae for best range

> 4.6 Rotator Cuffs - try to get back of hand/lower arm on ground.

Appendix F – Exercise List

Body	Exercise Type	Ref	Exercise Name
Arms	Triceps Extensions	A11	Cable Centre Parting
Arms	Triceps Extensions	A12	Barbell Lying Extension
Arms	Triceps Extensions	A13	Dumbbell Overhead Extension
Arms	Triceps Pushdowns	A21	Short Bar Pushdown
Arms	Triceps Pushdowns	A22	Rope Pushdown
Arms	Triceps Pushdowns	A23	Cable Road Drill
Arms	Triceps Others	A31	Seated Tricep Dip Machine
Arms	Triceps Others	A32	Cable Reverse Grip Pulldown
Arms	Triceps Others	A33	Cable Crossdown
Arms	Biceps Free Weights	A41	Seated Alternate Dumbbell Curl
Arms	Biceps Free Weights	A42	Cross-body Hammer Curl
Arms	Biceps Free Weights	A43	Standing Barbell Curl
Arms	Biceps Free Weights	A44	Concentration Curl
Arms	Biceps Free Weights	A45	Dumbbell Preacher Curl
Arms	Biceps Free Weights	A46	Barbell Preacher Curl
Arms	Biceps Free Weights	A47	Standing Alternate Dumbbell Curl
Arms	Biceps Free Weights	A48	Hammer Curl Bar
Arms	Biceps Machine	A51	Bicep Curl Machine
Arms	Biceps Machine	A52	Short Bar Cable Curl
Arms	Biceps Machine	A53	Standing High Cable Curl
Arms	Forearms	A61	Dumbbell Wrist Curl
Arms	Forearms	A62	Dumbbell Reverse Wrist Curl
Arms	Forearms	A63	Low Cable Reverse Curl
Arms	Triceps Finisher	A71	Tricep Dip
Back	Upper Back Rows	B11	Dumbbell Upright Row

Back	Upper Back Rows	B12	Cable Upright Row
Back	Upper Back Rows	B13	Barbell Upright Row
Back	Upper Back Rows	B14	Smith Machine Upright Row
Back	Upper Back Shrugs	B21	Dumbbell Vertical Shrug
Back	Upper Back Shrugs	B22	Cable Vertical Shrug
Back	Upper Back Shrugs	B23	Dumbbell Rotating Shrug
Back	Upper Back Shrugs	B24	Hexagonal Bar Shrug
Back	Mid Back Rows	B31	Seated Row Machine Neutral Grip
Back	Mid Back Rows	B32	Seated Low Cable Row
Back	Mid Back Rows	B33	Single Arm Dumbbell Row
Back	Mid Back Rows	B34	T-Bar Row
Back	Wide-Grip Pulls	B41	Lat Pulldown Vertical
Back	Wide-Grip Pulls	B42	Lat Pulldown Leanback
Back	Wide-Grip Pulls	B43	Fixed-path Pulldown Machine
Back	Narrow-Grip Pulls	B51	Close-grip Pull-up
Back	Narrow-Grip Pulls	B52	Close Under-grip Pulldown
Back	Narrow-Grip Pulls	B53	Close Neutral-grip Pulldown
Back	Lower Back	B61	Lumbar Extension Machine
Back	Lower Back	B62	Swiss Ball Lumbar Extension
Back	Lower Bac	B63	Incline Lumbar Extension
Back	Back Finisher	B71	Wide-grip Pullup
Chest	Upper Chest Press	C11	Smith Machine Incline Press
Chest	Upper Chest Press	C12	Single Arm Incline Cable Press
Chest	Upper Chest Press	C13	Incline Dumbbell Press
Chest	Upper Chest Press	C14	Incline Barbell Press
Chest	Upper Chest Press	C15	Incline Press Machine
Chest	Mid Chest Press	C21	Seated Chest Press Machine
Chest	Mid Chest Press	C22	Flat Bench Barbell Press
Chest	Mid Chest Press	C23	Flat Bench Dumbbell Press
Chest	Mid Chest Press	C24	Smith Machine Flat Press
Chest	Mid Chest Press	C25	Flat Bench Machine Press
Chest	Upper Chest Fly	C31	Pec Fly Machine High-grip
Chest	Upper Chest Fly	C32	Low Wide Incline Cable Fly
Chest	Upper Chest Fly	C33	Incline Dumbbell Fly
Chest	Upper Chest Fly	C34	Low Narrow Incline Cable Fly

Chest	Upper Chest Fly	C35	Standing Wide Low Cable Fly
Chest	Mid Chest Fly	C41	Pec Fly Machine Mid-grip
Chest	Mid Chest Fly	C42	Standing Cable Fly
Chest	Mid Chest Fly	C43	Flat Bench Dumbbell Fly
Chest	Mid Chest Fly	C44	Wide Cable Fly
Chest	Lower Chest	C51	Standing Narrow High Cable Fly
Chest	Lower Chest	C52	Decline Barbell Press
Chest	Lower Chest	C53	Decline Dumbbell Press
Chest	Lower Chest	C54	Standing Wide High Cable Fly
Chest	Lower Chest	C55	Decline Dumbbell Fly
Chest	Chest Pullovers	C61	Single Dumbbell Pullover
Chest	Chest Pullovers	C62	Double Dumbbell Pullover
Chest	Chest Pullovers	C63	Barbell Pullover
Chest	Chest Finisher	C71	Push Up
Deltoids	Shoulder Press	D11	Forward Grip Dumbbell Press
Deltoids	Shoulder Press	D12	Shoulder Press Machine
Deltoids	Shoulder Press	D13	Rotational Grip Dumbbell Press
Deltoids	Shoulder Press	D14	Standing Barbell Press
Deltoids	Shoulder Raise	D21	Front Cable Raise
Deltoids	Shoulder Raise	D22	Front Barbell Raise
Deltoids	Shoulder Raise	D23	Seated Alternate Dumbbell Raise
Deltoids	Lateral Side Raise	D31	Leaning Cable Raise
Deltoids	Lateral Side Raise	D32	Lateral Raise Machine
Deltoids	Lateral Side Raise	D33	Standing DB Lateral Raise – Straight
Deltoids	Lateral Side Raise	D34	Standing DB Lateral Raise – Bent
Deltoids	Rear Delt Machine	D41	Reverse Cable Crossover
Deltoids	Rear Delt Machine	D42	Rope Nose Pulls
Deltoids	Rear Delt Machine	D43	Seated Row Machine - Top Grip
Deltoids	Rear Delt Machine	D44	Rear Delt Fly Machine
Deltoids	Rear Delt Machine	D45	Prone Rear Delt Fly Machine
Deltoids	Rear Delt Free	D51	Pronated Rear Delt Dumbbell Fly
Deltoids	Rear Delt Free	D52	Incline Bench Rear Delt Fly
Deltoids	Rear Delt Free	D53	Seated Rear Delt Dumbbell Touch
Deltoids	Rotator Cuff	D61	Cable Internal Rotator Cuff
Deltoids	Rotator Cuff	D62	Lying Dumbbell Lateral Rotation

Deltoids	Rotator Cuff	D63	Lying Dumbbell Vertical Rotation
Deltoids	Shoulder Finisher	D71	Standing Barbell Press
Legs	Extensions + Lunges	L11	Leg Extension Machine
Legs	Extensions + Lunges	L12	Dumbbell Returning Lunge
Legs	Extensions + Lunges	L13	Dumbbell Walking Lunge
Legs	Hamstrings	L21	Seated Hamstring Curl
Legs	Hamstrings	L22	Lying Hamstring Curl
Legs	Hamstrings	L23	Barbell Stiff-leg Deadlift
Legs	Hamstrings	L24	Single-leg Bench Hips Raise
Legs	Hamstrings	L25	Swiss Ball Hips Raise
Legs	Hamstrings	L26	Hamstrings on Leg Press Machine
Legs	Machine Press	L31	Cradle Leg Press Machine
Legs	Machine Press	L32	Sled Leg Press Machine
Legs	Machine Press	L33	Seat-move Leg Press Machine
Legs	Machine Press	L34	Footplate-move Leg Press Machine
Legs	Squats	L41	Back Squat
Legs	Squats	L42	Smith Machine Squat
Legs	Squats	L43	Sumo Squat
Legs	Squats	L44	Hack Squat
Legs	Squats	L45	Goblet Squat
Legs	Straight Leg Calf	L51	Calf on Leg Press Machine
Legs	Straight Leg Calf	L52	Standing Calf Dumbbell Raise
Legs	Straight Leg Calf	L53	Rotary Calf Machine
Legs	Straight Leg Calf	L54	Standing Calf Raise Machine
Legs	Bent Leg Calf	L61	Seated Calf Raise Machine
Legs	Bent Leg Calf	L62	Seated Calf Dumbbells Raise
Legs	Bent Leg Calf	L63	Calf on Leg Extension Machine
Legs	Leg Finisher	L71	Toe Taps + Heel Raises
Mid	Upper Abs	M11	Decline Forwards Sit-up
Mid	Upper Abs	M12	Legs-supported Forward Crunch
Mid	Upper Abs	M13	Seated Ab Machine
Mid	Upper Abs	M14	High Cable Pulldown
Mid	Upper Abs	M15	Dumbbell-assisted Sit-up
Mid	Upper Abs	M16	Dumbbell Overhead V-Crunch
Mid	Upper Abs	M17	Swiss Ball Forward Crunch

Mid	Upper Abs	M18	Floor Crunch
Mid	Lower Abs	M21	Incline Leg Raise
Mid	Lower Abs	M22	Seated Knee Pull
Mid	Lower Abs	M23	Supported Knee Lift
Mid	Lower Abs	M24	Supported Straight Leg Lift
Mid	Lower Abs	M25	Swiss Ball Lift
Mid	Lower Abs	M26	Forward Legs Swiss Roll
Mid	Lower Abs	M27	Floor Heart
Mid	Lower Abs	M28	Floor Leg Pull
Mid	Lower Abs	M29	Frogs Legs
Mid	Obliques	M31	Decline Twisting Crunch
Mid	Obliques	M32	Dumbbell Side Bends
Mid	Obliques	M33	Horizontal Cable Rotation
Mid	Obliques	M34	Sideways Knee Lift
Mid	Obliques	M35	Twisting Legs Swiss Roll
Mid	Obliques	M36	Swiss Ball Rotating Crunch
Mid	Obliques	M37	Broomstick Twist
Mid	Obliques	M38	Bicycle Crunch
Mid	Obliques	M39	Torso Twist Machine
Mid	Core Stability	M41	Front Plank
Mid	Core Stability	M42	Alternating Plank Kickback
Mid	Core Stability	M43	Swiss Ball Bridge
Mid	Core Stability	M44	Swiss Ball Rolling Bridge
Mid	Core Stability	M45	Suspended Superman
Mid	Core Stability	M46	Alternating Superman Raises
Mid	Core Stability	M51	Side Plank
Mid	Core Stability	M52	Side Plank Leg Raise

Appendix G – Daily Data Sheet Format

In the example on the next page, you can see that the previous week had been very good on the water objective (7 days out of 7), and the least good performer was amount of fats consumed, hitting the objective on 2 days out of 7.

There is also a total for the week (40 objectives achieved out of 70). The final column is the type of training undertaken on that day, from the three types described in Chapter 17 – Weights, Core or Stretching.

The data from this sheet can be used to adjust behaviour for the following week. Although, with a loss of 0.6kg on the average calculation and bodyfat percentage also down, nothing needs to change at this point to keep on track for this example user. However, it may be increasing the number of objectives achieved would cause an increase in the rate of decrease of weight and/or bodyfat percentage.

Date	Weight	Wt-Ave	BF %	BF-ave	Kcal	Protein	Sugars	Fats	SatFats	Hours	Water	Cardio	Steps	Train	Type
1/1/20	80.0	80.0	23.4	23.4	1	0	0	0	0	0	1	0	1	1	S
2/1/20	80.0	80.0	23.1	23.3	0	1	1	0	0	1	1	1	0	1	C
3/1/20	79.5	79.8	24.0	23.5	1	1	0	1	0	1	1	1	1	0	
4/1/20	79.1	79.7	23.8	23.6	0	0	1	1	0	1	1	0	0	1	W
5/1/20	79.3	79.6	23.3	23.5	1	1	1	0	1	0	1	0	1	0	
6/1/20	79.1	79.5	22.9	23.4	0	1	1	0	0	1	1	1	0	1	S
7/1/20	78.8	79.4	22.7	23.3	1	1	0	0	1	0	1	0	1	0	
					4	5	5	2	2	4	7	3	4	4	40
8/1/20	78.8	79.2	22.9	23.2	0	1	0	1	1	1	0	1	0	1	C
9/1/20															

Appendix H – No-Gym Resistance Workout

Here is my 20:20 Workout, designed for those without access to a gym or on holiday. It's called the 20:20 as the workout contains 20 exercises, each of which has 20 repetitions. That may sound a lot, but it should take less than 20 minutes – another reason to call it 20:20.

The 20:20 Workout includes exercises for all major muscle groups plus abs, plus an element of cardio, and some optional recommended stretching and flexibility work at the end. The only equipment you need is a chair, a door with doorknobs either side, and a wall.

The exercises are grouped into 4 groups, each with 5 exercises:

1. Warm-up/Cardio,
2. Upper Body,
3. Lower Body,
4. Abs / Core.

I have chosen the exercises to be particularly applicable to the 50+ age group, nothing too difficult (so no one-arm handstands, for example), but hopefully a little bit challenging for most people. Most of the resistance exercises work multiple muscle groups – I have indicated the major muscle group worked by each exercise.

The target is 20 repetitions ('reps') or 20 seconds. But if you're new to it, start by attempting 10 repetitions. If you fail before this on any or all exercises, that's fine, make a note of the number you fail on, and try to do one closer to 20 next time. But always fail and stop doing that exercise at that point rather than continue to do an exercise with dodgy form. Take a few moments rest between each exercise, but not too long or you'll blow that 20 minutes.

For each exercise, a rep is once you have completed a movement and are back at the starting position. Note that within each rep within the upper body and lower body groups, there are two movements: the exertion phase, where you push or pull some weight against the force of gravity, and the returning phase, where gravity is taking the weight downwards.

Two of my favourite words in resistance training are 'Lower Slower' – you should resist gravity on this second phase, don't let gravity do the work. The returning phase should take twice as long as the exertion phase on average – say 4 seconds lowering following 2 second of the exertion phase.

And another favourite word is 'Exonex' – OK it's not a real word, I made it up – but it means Exhale on Exertion. So, breathe out as you push or pull the weight quickly, then breathe in as you lower slower.

Here are the 20 exercises, and this is where your 20 minutes starts. We start with some warm-up exercises that get the cardio system moving a little, and get you a little (or more) out of breath.

Warm-up/Cardio (5 exercises)

High Knees Running:

Running on the spot, getting those knees as high as possible in front of you – ideally past the point of the upper leg being horizontal. A rep is once you have lifted both right and left legs. So, for your initial 10-rep pattern, you lift each leg 10 times.

Full Star Jumps:

Stand upright with hands by your sides. Jump up and spread your legs while jumping, so that when you land, your feet are apart, ideally wider than shoulder width apart. While jumping, raise your arms in a wide arc so that, when you land, your hands are touching vertically over your head. Try to keep arms straight throughout. Reverse the movement back to the starting position.

Squat Jumps:

Start standing upright, feet close together and arms by your sides. Squat down as low as you can go, drop your hands so your fingertips are touching the floor in front of your toes. This is the starting position. Then jump up a high as you can, reaching overhead with your hands as far up as you can. The come back down (gravity does the first bit) to the starting position, touching the floor with your fingertips. Wait a fraction second before the next rep.

Mountain Climbs:

Start face down on the floor, weight on hands and toes, arms straight. Bring one foot forward so that the knee on the side is right by the chest. This is the starting position. Now quickly push that leg down, and bring the other one up, so that the positions are reversed. Lift both feet off the floor briefly as they move (not dragging along the floor). Pause for a fraction of a second, then reverse the movement back to the starting position, where you pause again before the next rep. 10 reps is 10 times bringing each leg forward alternately – so there are 20 moves in your initial 10 rep pattern.

Low Burpees:

Similar to the Mountain Climbs, but both feet move in the same direction at once. Start face down on the floor, weight on hands and toes, arms straight. Bring both feet forward, so that the knees are right by the chest. Now quickly push both legs down to the starting position. Lift both feet off the floor briefly as they move (not dragging along the floor). Wait a fraction of a second before the next rep.

You should be well warmed up by now, heart rate appropriately elevated, ready to move on to the next group – 5 exercises for the upper body.

Upper Body (5 exercises)

Press Ups: (Chest)

There are many ways to do a press up, but I like the simplest one. Face down, body flat on the floor, hands flat on the floor alongside shoulders and fingers forwards. Press up while exhaling until elbows are almost locked, and then lower slower. Stop when any part of your upper body is very nearly touching the floor. Keep the body straight as a plank from the heels upwards throughout the movement. If it's too difficult, the easier variant keeps the knees on the floor as well as toes, and the plank goes from the knees up the body. And if that's too hard, try it leaning up against a wall. Alternatively, if you want to make it more difficult than the basic, elevate the feet by having the toes resting on a step.

Overhand Pulls: (Back)

Find a door with a handle on both sides. Hotel bathroom is my favourite. Stand facing the edge of the open door, holding each handle in an overhand grip. Move your feet forward, alongside the bottom of the door, and sink backwards so that your arms are straight. This is the starting position. Then, with elbows going outwards (not downwards), pull yourself forwards as far as possible – which is usually when your head is about to hit the door edge. Hold for a fraction of a second, feeling a bit or a squeeze in the upper back, then lower slower back to the starting position. Keep the body straight throughout, don't lead forwards. Remember Lower Slower and Exonex. And please don't pull the door off its hinges – try a couple of lightweight pulls the first time you do this to get a sense if the door fixings can take it! Putting the feet further forward makes this a harder and better exercise. You can use a horizontal bar instead if you have one to use.

Underhand Pulls: (Biceps)

Find a door with a handle on both sides. Stand facing the edge of the open door, holding each handle in an underhand grip. Move your feet forward, alongside the bottom of the door, and sink backwards so that your arms are straight. This is the starting position. Then, with elbows going downwards (not outwards), pull yourself forwards as far as possible – which is usually when your head is about to hit the door edge. Hold for a fraction of a second, feeling a slight squeeze in the biceps, then back to the starting position. Remember Lower Slower and Exonex. Keep the body straight throughout, don't lean forwards. Putting the feet further forward makes this a harder and better exercise (but increases the pressure on those hinges!). You can use a horizontal bar instead if you have one to use.

Tricep Dips: (Triceps)

Find a chair that is stable – a dining chair is ideal. Wheels are a no-no. Sit on the edge of the chair, hands gripping the outer edge of the arms of the chair – or gripping the front edge of the chair if the chair has no arms. With legs straight, and heels on the floor, move forward slightly so your weight is on your arms and heels only. Then lower through your arms as the elbows flare outwards. When you can go no further, push back up to the starting position. Lower Slower than the push back up, and Exonex. If there is any instability in the chair position, try pushing it up against the wall. Make this easier by making the chair higher and vice versa. Make it extra hard by raising the feet on to something solid.

Shoulder Walls: (Shoulders)

Stand upright facing a wall, away from the wall by the approximate length of your upper body. Tilt forward at the waist so your back is horizontal and with your hands on the wall, alongside your head, fingers upwards. You should be looking downwards, with the top of your head very close to the wall. This is the starting position. From here push with your hands so your upper body moves backwards – don't move your feet. The ideal end position has your back and arms in a straight line – horizontal. Reverse back to the starting position. Make it much more difficult, if you want to, by doing it one arm at a time (sorry, have to double the reps if you do this).

By now, you are half way through and should be sometime around 10 minutes into it (obviously much longer the first couple of times as you are getting used to it and still reading the instructions). Good news is if you've done the full 20 reps per exercise, you've done 200 reps in total – a great first half.

Lower Body (5 exercises)

Lunges: (Quadriceps)

Start by standing upright, feet close together facing forwards, and arms by your sides. Each rep has three phases – firstly, place one leg on the floor ahead by bending the knee – keep the back leg straight and both feet facing forwards. Ideally the upper part of the stretched-out leg is parallel to the floor. Secondly, sink downwards so that your rear knee touches the ground (or gets very close to it). Thirdly, push back up from the front leg so that, in one motion, you are back at the starting position. Do it all again with the other leg. Try to keep the back vertical and head facing straight on throughout. Lower Slower doesn't really apply, but the exertion is on the third phase, so this should be the exhale point. And yes, you can hold on to something for stability, but not to be weight-bearing. We count one rep here as the movement on either leg, so the set of 10 reps is 5 per side alternately. Make it more difficult by lengthening the stride of the step forwards.

One-leg Squats: (Quadriceps)

Stand with one leg on behind you with that foot up on a chair. Lower down by bending the standing leg as far as feels right, then return to the starting position. Then the same on the other side. Feel free to hold on to something for stability, but not to be weight-bearing. We count one rep here as the movement on either leg, so the set of 10 reps is 5 per side – do all one side first, then the other. Make it more difficult by lengthening the stride of the step forwards, and sinking a bit further. Also known as Bulgarian squats, don't know why, if you do, can you let me know?

Wide Squats: (Hamstrings and quads)

Stand with feet fairly wide apart – more than shoulder width apart, hands by your sides, feet forwards or slightly outwards. Keeping the back as straight and vertical as possible, and the head up, bend at the knees and drop the hands in front of you so that the fingertips touch the floor – if you can't reach the floor, go as far as you feel is good. Keep looking straight in front the whole time - this helps keep the back straight. Then return to the starting position. This is made more difficult by getting more of your hand and wrist to touch the floor.

Stair Rocks: (Calves)

Stand on the edge of a stair, holding on to the handrail, weight on the front part of the feet with heels hanging over the edge. Hinge upwards and downwards to the maximum range of movement. One up and one down is one rep. Do the downward movement particularly slowly, as the Achilles Tendon is vulnerable to sudden movements such as this.

Hip Raises: (Glutes and Hamstrings)

Lie on the floor with upper legs vertical, lower legs horizontal resting on a chair. Right angles at the knee and hip. Using your hamstrings and glutes (not pushing with your hands), lift your hips off the floor so that your torso and upper legs become a straight line – probably 30 degrees or so to the ground. Lower slower but don't quite get the hips back on the ground before doing the next rep. Make it much harder by doing one leg at a time, with the non-exercised leg pointing up, parallel to the other thigh.

Abs/Core (5 exercises)

Floor Crunches: (Upper Abs)

Lie on the floor, legs bent with your knees at the top of a pyramid. Then, with hands by your hips, curl upwards a short distance, then down again under slow control. Lower slower. Try to keep the feet on the floor, and don't rock. Do go so far upwards that it is easy - keep the motion of the head in a vertical plane, not horizontal. And don't touch the floor with your shoulders between each rep.

Straight Leg Lifts: (Lower Abs)

Lie flat on the floor, feet together. Then, keeping legs straight, raise legs as far as possible then bring them down again towards (but not quite touching) the floor. Don't add swing or momentum, and keep the hips on the floor. If this is too hard, bend your knees so the lower legs remain parallel to the ground.

Bicycle Crunches: (Obliques)

Lie on the floor, legs straight out in front of you, hands at your temples. Lift your feet and legs slightly off the ground, then bring your right knee towards your chest, at the same time extending and twisting your upper left side so that your left elbow touches the inside of your right knee. Return more slowly to the start position, then do the same on the other side. One rep is a complete left and right cycle - so there are forty movements in total.

Front Plank: (Core)

Lie flat on the floor face down, then raise yourself such that you are resting on your elbows and toes. The upper arms are vertical, the lower arms are on the floor. The body is to remain flat in this raised position, no sagging at the middle – Plank-like, in fact. 20 seconds holding this position.

Side Planks: (Core)

Lie on the floor on your right side, then raise then raise yourself such that you are resting on your right elbow and side of your right foot. The upper part of the right arm is vertical, the lower part of the right arm is on the floor. Left leg lies on top of the right one, and left arm is lying on the body. The body is to remain flat in this raised position, no sagging at the middle – Plank-like, in fact. 10 seconds holding this position, then the same for the other side.

That's it – 20 exercises, each of which has 20 reps or takes 20 seconds, and all over in 20 minutes. And you can do this every alternate day – and no need to go anywhere near a gym.

Appendix I – Nutrition Calculation Approach

The calories, correctly called kilocalories (Kcal), of any food or drink is the amount of energy supplied by that food item. The definition of a calorie is the amount of energy needed to raise the temperature of 1kg of water through 1 degree C.

Energy exists in all foods, and foods are made up of macronutrients. Every gram of protein or carbohydrates supplies 4 calories (some authorities say 3.75) and every gram of fat provides 9 calories. Although not referenced here, every gram of alcohol gives 7 calories and fibre supplies either 2 calories or zero, depending on viewpoint. I tend to ignore fibre as the calories from fibre are minimally absorbed by the body and have a negligible effect on blood sugar.

Here is an explanation of the maths behind calories and grams. I am looking at the 30% of calories from for protein sources, and 30% of calories from fat sources that I suggest, and using 2000 total kcal as an example:

1. 30% of calories from protein means 600 calories from protein, and at 4 calories per gram that gives 150 grams.

2. 30% of calories from fat means 600 calories from fat, and at 9 calories per gram that gives 67 grams.

3. The remaining 40% of calories will come from carbs, which means 800 calories from carbs, and at 4 calories per gram that gives 200 grams. You don't measure carbs on this plan.

4. The opinions on sugar vary, and I have selected 13.4% of all calories to come from sugar. That means 268 calories from sugar, which at 4 calories per gram (as sugar is a carb) is 67g. This is also the same number as total fats, making it easier to remember.

5. The opinions on saturated fats also vary, and I have selected 9% of all calories to come from saturates. That means 180 calories from saturates, which at 9 calories per gram (as sugar is a carb) is 20g.

This can be shown as a table, similar to a nutrition panel on a food item:

	Kcals	Kcals	= grams	= % of total Kcal
Total	100%	2000		
Protein	30%	600	150	7.50%
Carbs	40%	600	200	10.00%
of which sugars:	13.4%	268	67	3.35%
Fats	30%	600	67	3.35%
of which saturates:	9%	180	20	1.00%

The final column is not of any real value (as it is dividing grams into a calorie number), except as a short cut in the computation. To calculate the number of grams of a nutrient needed for success in accordance with these principles simply multiply the overall calories per day by this factor. Calculating 3.35% of 2000 gives 67 – the grams of both sugar and saturated fats from a 2000/Kcal day plan.

Appendix J – Sample Day Nutrition

	Kcal	Protein	Sugars	Fats	Sat Fats	Carbs
Oats 65g	244	7	0	5	1	39
Protein Shake 25g	100	19	1	2	1	2
Mixed Nuts 25g	154	5	1	13	1	2
Berries 0.5 Cup	42	1	7	0	0	11
	540	32	10	21	4	53
Spag Carbonara	324	20	6	5	3	49
Mixed Veg	46	3	4	1	0	6
Yoghurt	83	8	10	1	0	11
	453	30	20	6	3	66
Protein Shake 50g	200	38	1	4	2	4
Apple	52	0	10	0	0	14
	252	38	11	4	2	18
Protein Bar	214	22	1	9	5	14
Beef + Ale Dinner	405	63	12	9	4	17
Mixed Veg	46	3	4	1	0	6
Choc Mousse	86	4	9	2	1	14
	537	69	25	12	5	37
Totals	1996	192	67	51	18	187

Numbers do not compute exactly due to rounding and differing methods of calculation used by suppliers.

Overall carb numbers are included for completeness, not because they are referenced by the plan.

Appendix Z – Zaremba's Quotes

Here are some of my favourite phrases to do with fitness. I believe I coined them all; although it's possible that some might have entered my consciousness subliminally from elsewhere first!

Some are a play on words, some a little humorous, some neither – but they all have a point in their message. If you've read the entire book, you'll have come across most of them already.

- Add years to your life, and life to your years.

- Bored or depressed? Calories for comfort are not the solution. Food is not a hug.

- Count the reps, and make the reps count.

- Exonex – Exhale on exertion.

- Fitness-up and fatness-down.

- Getting fit is Elementary – Eat Less, Exercise More, Extend Nights, Towards A Renewed You.

- Getting fit isn't rocket science – it's rocket salad.

- I workout so I can go out.

- If there's something you really want to do, you'll find a way of doing it. If there's something you really don't want to do, you'll find an excuse.

- If you can measure it, you can improve it.

- If you see any red, take something instead.

- It's never too late to start something new.

- Lower slower.

- Plan your eats; then eat your plan.

- QNQ – Quality, Not Quantity.

- The DROP law – the Diminishing Returns Of Pleasure.

- The number one factor in determining the overall success or not of your fitness plans is your ability to prioritise your long-term wants over your short-term wants. Do you want to live a long, healthy, fit and happy life, or do you want to eat that creamy jammy doughnut?

- There are 168 hours in a week. As a trainer, I see you for one of those hours. The success of your fitness journey doesn't depend on that one hour; it depends on what you do in the 167.

- What gets written, gets done.

- You're not on a diet; you're eating in accordance with your lifestyle.

REFERENCES

Note that Upper Case where shown is important in most of these links.

---

[1] Videos of exercises: www.bitly.com/ChrisExerciseVideos

[2] Personal Training: www.bitly.com/ChrisPT

[3] My website: www.FitnessOverFIfty.co.uk

[4] Personal Training: www.bitly.com/ChrisPT

[5] Fit Happens + ABC7 Systems: www.bitly.com/ChrisWorkoutSystems

[6] Nutrition and recipe books: www.bitly.com/ChrisNutritionPlans

[7] YouTube channel: www.bitly.com/ChrisVideos

[8] Monthly club Fit Club 50: www.bitly.com/OverviewOfFitClub50

[9] Fat to Fit at 50 documentary: www.bitly.com/FTFDocumentary

[10] MarlowFM Radio: www.MarlowFM.co.uk

[11] Fit Happens TV, both series: www.Fit-Happens.co.uk

[12] The Fit Happens podcast: www.anchor.fm/ChrisZaremba

[13] Generation Challenge: www.bitly.com/GenerationChallenge

[14] Dan Wynes site: www.DanWynesFitness.com

[15] Generation Revenge: www.bitly.com/GenerationRevenge

[16] Safety bar for squats: www.bitly.com/SafetyBarForSquats

[17] Life After Fifty: www.bitly.com/ChrisLifeAfterFifty

[18] Stage One Workout: www.bitly.com/StageOneWorkout

[19] Treadmill Introduction: www.bitly.com/TreadmillIntro

[20] Cross-Trainer Introduction: www.bitly.com/CrossTrainerIntro

[21] Workout without gym: www.bitly.com/WorkoutWithoutGym

[22] Calories used calculator: www.bitly.com/CaloriesUsedCalculator

[23] Cross-Trainer Introduction: www.bitly.com/CrossTrainerIntro

[24] Treadmill Introduction: www.bitly.com/TreadmillIntro

[25] Exercise videos: www.bitly.com/ChrisExerciseVideos

[26] Personal Training: www.bitly.com/ChrisPT

[27] Exercise Videos: www.bitly.com/ChrisExerciseVideos

[28] Typical Stretches: www.bitly.com/ChrisStretches

[29] Stage One Workout: www.bitly.com/StageOneWorkout

Printed in Great Britain
by Amazon

60446643R00203